Navigating the Caregiving Journey

A Practical Guide to Support Systems,
Self-care and Balance

ANDREA
ENTWISTLE

First published by Ultimate World Publishing 2025

ISBN

Paperback: 978-1-923425-39-2
Ebook: 978-1-923425-40-8

Cover design: Ultimate World Publishing
Layout and typesetting: Ultimate World Publishing
Editor: Alex Floyd-Douglass

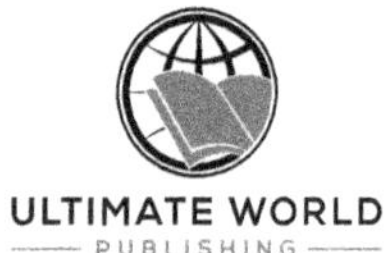

Ultimate World Publishing
Diamond Creek,
Victoria Australia 3089
www.writeabook.com.au

Disclaimer

This book provides general information, strategies and insights based on personal and professional caregiving experiences. It is intended for informational purposes only and should not be considered medical, legal or financial advice. Readers are encouraged to consult qualified professionals for specific advice tailored to their individual circumstances.

While every effort has been made to ensure the accuracy of the information provided, neither the author nor *A1 Quality Care* shall be held responsible for any decisions made or actions taken based on the content of this book. The author does not accept any liability for errors, omissions or outcomes resulting from the application of the information presented.

Any references to support services, government funding or external resources are subject to change and readers should verify details with the appropriate authorities.

The stories shared in this book are based on real experiences; however, to respect privacy and confidentiality, all names and identifying details have been changed. Some examples are also illustrative for educational purposes.

By reading this book, you acknowledge that the author and publisher are not responsible for any consequences arising from your use of the information herein.

Testimonials

"*Navigating the Caregiving Journey* is a heartfelt and empowering story of caregiving from every angle. As both a mother of four children with different needs – one of whom requires round-the-clock care – and someone who works in a caregiving role and as a business manager, this novel truly hit home for me. It beautifully portrays the complexities of caregiving, shedding light on the emotional and physical toll it takes while reminding us of the vital importance of self-care.

For those of us in caregiving roles, it's easy to forget that we need care, too. The author's message is clear: Without taking time to nurture ourselves, we can't provide the support and attention our loved ones need. As a mother, I've felt the weight of this truth firsthand. This novel was a powerful reminder that self-care isn't a luxury – it's a necessity. Only when we care for ourselves can we be fully present for those we love and care for.

Whether you're a mother, a caregiver, or someone in a support role, this book resonates with anyone who understands the balancing act of caring for others while making sure you don't lose sight of your own well-being. It's an empowering and essential read for anyone on this journey."

**Cheri Murphy,
A Mother and Primary Caregiver**

"Finally, *Navigating the Caregiving Journey* is a book that not only simplifies the complexities of a carer's role but also validates the overwhelming emotions we often experience. Thank you, Andrea! I could put the book down and pick it back up without feeling the need to restart a chapter, making it truly accessible in my busy life – and the worksheets are an absolute godsend.

As the primary kinship carer for my two granddaughters, who have complex disabilities and trauma-related challenges, this book has given me a practical framework to implement strategies that ease my overwhelm. At last – something that truly helps!"

Sharon Le Fort,
A Kinship Carer

Dedication

<hr>

This book is dedicated to all of you who are on the challenging journey of caregiving. To the readers who tirelessly strive to provide love, support and care for their loved ones, this book is a tribute to your unwavering strength, compassion and resilience.

May it serve as a guide, a source of comfort and a reminder that you are not alone on this path. Your dedication and commitment to the well-being of others inspire us all.

I also need to acknowledge my beautiful mum, whose boundless love, nurturing spirit and unwavering presence shaped me into the person I am today. Losing her was the deepest heartache I've ever known, yet her life continues to inspire every word and every page of this work.

Mum, you were not only my greatest teacher but my dearest friend and your grace still echoes in every corner of my soul. I love you beyond measure and hold onto the hope that one day, we will meet again.

Until then, your legacy lives on in every part of me.

Contents

Preface

I never imagined I would find myself on this journey, yet here I am – just like you – learning, adapting and navigating the ever-changing world of caregiving. Whether your path began suddenly or unfolded over time, one thing is certain: caregiving transforms us in ways we never expected.

As a professional support worker, I see caregivers every day – people who are exhausted yet devoted, overwhelmed yet determined, stretched thin yet still giving. I've listened to their stories, their frustrations, their hopes and their fears. I understand the invisible weight they carry because I, too, have walked this path – not just professionally but personally.

My own caregiving journey was shaped by my mum, a woman I loved fiercely and cared for deeply. When she became unwell, I stepped into the role of her caregiver, facing the emotional and physical demands that so many of us know all too well.

Then, when COVID-19 arrived, the world changed – and so did our reality. The pandemic didn't just take lives; it reshaped the way we lived, loved and grieved. Losing Mum during that time was an experience unlike any other. The isolation, the fear, the helplessness – it left an imprint on me that I will carry forever.

It also deepened my understanding of caregiving. I realised that beyond the practical tasks, there is an emotional toll that often goes unspoken. Caregivers don't just need systems and strategies; they need support, community and permission to care for themselves, too.

This book is the guide I wish I had. It's not just about managing the day-to-day tasks; it's about creating a caregiving system that works for you, one that lightens the load and helps you reclaim a sense of balance. It's about building a network of support, finding ways to care for yourself and ensuring that, amid the giving, you don't lose sight of who you are. This book is designed to be gentle with you, too – read it gradually, return to it when needed, or skip ahead to chapters that speak to your current season.

Throughout these pages, you'll find real-life stories, practical strategies and workbook activities. In my experience, the most valuable workbooks are the ones you can print and write in by hand.

In order to download the PDF version of the workbooks, go to www. a1-quality-care.com/book. You will need to fill out the form completely, including the code for the PDF document download: 'Caregiver23'

Beyond that, you'll find reassurance that you're not alone. Caregiving can feel isolating, but together, we can shift the narrative – from simply surviving to truly thriving.

Wherever you are on this journey, I hope this book offers you the support, guidance and encouragement you need. Take what resonates, apply what helps and always remember: **you matter, too.**

With warmth and understanding,
Andrea

PART 1:
THE BEGINNING
Stepping Into Caregiving

Caregiving has long been a natural part of family life, but with more care shifting into the home, loved ones now step into the role without hesitation – or preparation.

What begins as an act of love soon becomes an emotional and physical rollercoaster, demanding more than expected. This section explores where caregiving began, how it has evolved and how to navigate the challenges of stepping up while finding balance and support.

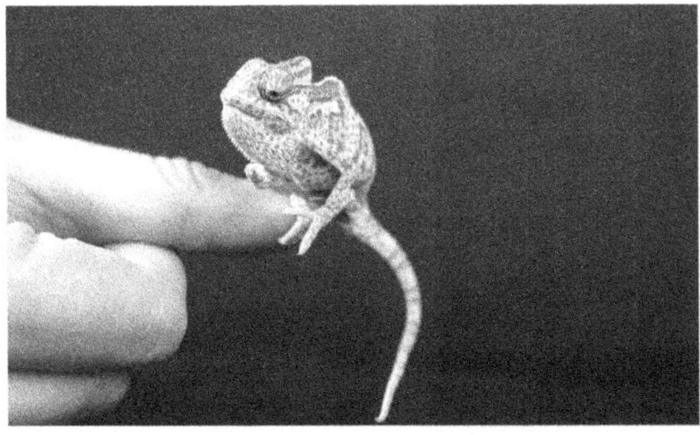

"A newborn chameleon doesn't yet know the colours it can become. With gentle guidance and time, it learns to blend, to adapt and to protect itself in a world it's only just discovering."
(Andrea Entwistle)

INTRODUCTION

The Shifting Landscape of Caregiving

Caregiving has always been a profound act of love and devotion. Historically, care for our ageing parents, disabled family members and loved ones recovering from illness was entrusted to institutions – nursing homes, hospitals and respite facilities.

For decades, this was considered the gold standard. Families believed professional care in these settings would offer the highest level of security and expertise, ensuring their loved ones were safeguarded within structured routines. Yet, there was an undeniable truth – no institution could ever replace the warmth, familiarity and love of home.

Over time, a radical shift began. A powerful movement emerged – one that championed dignity, independence and quality of life over institutional convenience. Families recognised that keeping loved ones at home, within familiar surroundings, led to greater emotional well-being, sharper cognitive function and an overall sense of belonging. Advances in home support services, government funding and innovative community-based programs empowered families to reclaim caregiving, offering an alternative to the sterile, regimented environment of institutional care. This transformation has granted countless individuals the right to age, heal and thrive at home, enveloped in love and personal connection.

However, this shift has placed an enormous responsibility on the shoulders of the primary caregiver – us. The reality is that keeping a loved one at home is both a privilege and a profound challenge. Most of us don't enter caregiving as professionals; we are simply devoted family members, partners or friends who rise to the occasion. And yet, from the moment we take on this role, we must embody resilience, resourcefulness and unshakable determination.

One of the greatest hurdles is navigating the complex and often overwhelming world of support services, funding and home care strategies. Unlike traditional caregiving models where trained professionals dictated routines, we – family caregivers – must now become the masterminds of an entire caregiving ecosystem. We immerse ourselves in research, battle bureaucracy, advocate tirelessly and construct systems that will ensure the best possible life for our loved ones. We are not just caregivers; we are warriors of love and champions of dignity.

Beyond the practical side of caregiving, there is the immense emotional and financial impact. Many of us have made life-altering sacrifices – scaling back careers, relinquishing financial stability and reshaping our entire existence to prioritise the needs of our loved ones. The weight of this responsibility is immense and yet, we persevere. Why? Because we understand that no facility, no matter how well-equipped, can offer the boundless love, patience and commitment that we provide. We are the heartbeat of home-based care and our devotion changes lives in ways that statistics and policies will never fully capture.

This book is your roadmap, your survival guide and your source of unwavering encouragement. It is designed to empower you – to give you the strategies, tools and knowledge to navigate caregiving with confidence and clarity. Each chapter will tackle the most critical challenges you face, from establishing home care systems to building unbreakable support networks, conquering stress and fiercely protecting your own well-being.

I wrote this book because I have walked this path myself. Love is what led me here – an unshakable love for my mum that left no room for hesitation. When she needed care, I stepped forward, not as a trained professional but as a daughter determined to give her the dignity, comfort and love she deserved.

I know what it feels like to be thrown into caregiving without a map, trying to balance love and duty while holding onto fragments of your own life. I've felt the exhaustion that seeps into your bones, the relentless decision-making, the advocacy that feels like an uphill battle. And yet, amid the chaos, I have also experienced the profound beauty of caregiving – the quiet victories, the unspoken gratitude, the moments of deep connection that remind you why you keep going.

This book is the guide I wish I had when I started. It is filled with hard-earned lessons, practical tools and the reassurance that you are not alone. My hope is that within these pages, you will find clarity, strength and a renewed sense of purpose. Because caregiving is not just a role – it's an act of love, courage and resilience. And no matter how overwhelming it may feel at times, you are capable, you are resourceful and you are never walking this journey alone.

> *"Caring for others is an expression of the heart but caring for yourself is an act of survival."* (Unknown)

CHAPTER 1

The Emotional Rollercoaster

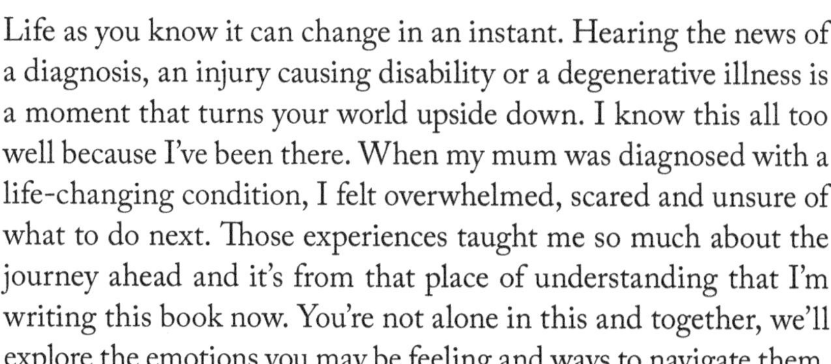

Life as you know it can change in an instant. Hearing the news of a diagnosis, an injury causing disability or a degenerative illness is a moment that turns your world upside down. I know this all too well because I've been there. When my mum was diagnosed with a life-changing condition, I felt overwhelmed, scared and unsure of what to do next. Those experiences taught me so much about the journey ahead and it's from that place of understanding that I'm writing this book now. You're not alone in this and together, we'll explore the emotions you may be feeling and ways to navigate them.

According to a study by the National Institute for Health Research, nearly 70% of carers experience significant anxiety within the first three months of adjusting to a diagnosis.
(National Institute for Health Research, Caregiver Burnout and Mental Health Study, 2022)

This is a common challenge and recognising your emotions is an important first step towards addressing it.

In this chapter, we will explore the emotional impact of caregiving and the journey that follows a life-changing diagnosis. Whether you are stepping into this role unexpectedly or have been on this path for some time, understanding the emotional landscape is essential. We will navigate the complexities of these feelings, offering insights into the challenges and strategies that can help you find strength and clarity.

Specifically, we will cover:

- The emotional rollercoaster and its impact on caregivers
- Recognising and processing emotions effectively
- The role of grief, fear, guilt and anger in the caregiving experience
- How a diagnosis affects not just the individual but the entire family dynamic
- The importance of open communication and emotional expression
- Strategies to build resilience and maintain emotional well-being
- Finding and creating support networks for both you and your loved one
- Practical steps to navigate uncertainty and regain a sense of control

This journey is deeply personal but you don't have to walk it alone. Let's begin.

Let's take a moment to focus on our emotions. After all, you might be thinking, 'I've got so much to do already – why add this?' But here's the thing: emotions are like a compass. They're guiding you, whether you realise it or not. Ignoring them can make things harder but understanding them can help you make better decisions, connect with others and even feel stronger in the long run.

Emotions are like your internal compass helping you figure out where to go when life feels overwhelming. Fear, for example, can nudge you to ask important questions or make a change you've been avoiding. Grief reminds you how much you value something that's changed or been lost. Even anger while it can feel all-consuming is often a sign that something in your life needs to shift. Instead of pushing these emotions aside try to see them as signals that are there to guide you.

When you bottle up your emotions, they don't just disappear. It's a bit like stuffing a suitcase until it's ready to burst – eventually, everything spills out and not in a good way. Suppressing your feelings can leave you feeling stressed, snappy or completely drained. But when you give those emotions a bit of room to breathe, you might find that they're not as overwhelming as they first seemed. Letting them out in a healthy way can be a huge relief.

Talking about what you're feeling can make a big difference, too. When you open up to someone you trust – a friend a loved one or even a professional – it helps them understand what you're going through. It can be scary to share but it's also a way to build stronger connections and let others support you. You don't have to face tough times alone and talking things out can make everything feel a bit more manageable.

Dealing with your emotions head-on isn't easy, but it's how you grow. Every time you take the time to understand what you're feeling and why, you become stronger and more resilient. It's like working a muscle – the more you practise the better you get. Over time, you'll build the confidence to face whatever life throws your way knowing you've got the tools to handle it.

My Journey with Mum

When I reflect on the importance of emotions, I can't help but think of my own journey with my mum. Her diagnosis was a turning point that reshaped not only her life but also ours as a family. It was as if the ground beneath us shifted leaving us to navigate unfamiliar territory filled with uncertainty and fear. The day we learned of her illness, I remember the weight of grief settling over me – not just for what she was facing, but for the future we had all envisioned slipping away.

She was only 64 and the thought of losing her so young felt unbearable. The years of togetherness we'd imagined – family holidays, laughter-filled gatherings and the milestones still to come – were suddenly overshadowed by the stark reality of her diagnosis. The idea that there would be no more Christmases with her at the heart of our celebrations, or that she would never meet the great-grandchild on the way, left an ache that has never truly faded.

For my mum, the diagnosis was more than just a personal loss – it brought about a professional reckoning, too. As a registered nurse, she had spent her career nurturing others back to health. She understood all too well the physical and emotional toll of caregiving a knowledge that once gave her purpose and pride. But as her illness progressed into the palliative stages, this same understanding added an extra layer of grief and fear. She was no longer the caregiver but the one in need of care; a role reversal that was deeply challenging for her to accept. Her identity so closely tied to being the one who provided strength and support now felt uncertain and fragile.

I saw how much she struggled with this shift. Her pride and independence which had defined her throughout her life were now tested in ways she never expected. Losing that sense of self – the nurse, the caregiver, the pillar of strength – was one of the hardest parts of her journey. It made me realise how closely our identity is tied to what we do and the roles we play. When those roles are taken away, it can feel like losing a part of ourselves.

For me, the emotional toll was immense. Fear gripped me as I worried about what the future held, not just for her but for all of us. I felt paralysed by grief, mourning the life she had planned and the things she might no longer experience. Guilt often crept in, too, as I second-guessed every decision and wondered if I was doing enough. And then there was anger – at the unfairness of the situation, at the lack of control and sometimes even at myself for not always knowing how to cope.

But over time, I learned to face these emotions rather than run from them. I realised that my feelings weren't wrong – they were human. They were a reflection of how much I cared. My mum's diagnosis, as devastating as it was, taught me the value of sitting with those emotions and allowing them to guide me. Fear pushed me to ask questions I might have avoided. Grief reminded me how deeply I valued her presence. Even anger, when I let myself feel it, revealed what needed to change in my approach to caregiving and my own well-being.

This journey taught me that emotions are not just challenges to overcome but signals of what matters most. It wasn't easy, but through acceptance and hope, I found strength I didn't know I had. And through it all, my mum's resilience and courage reminded me that even in the hardest times, there's room for connection love and growth.

Understanding Your Loved One's Journey and Their Emotions

A diagnosis doesn't just affect the person receiving it – it reshapes the entire family dynamic. As their abilities change, they may face losing their job, daily responsibilities or sense of independence, which can be a difficult adjustment. Relying on others for support can feel like a loss of control and emotions may run high as everyone adapts to the new reality. During this time, patience and open communication are essential. Expressing emotions honestly can help both of you navigate this transition with greater understanding and compassion.

For many, identity is deeply tied to their work, family role or self-reliance. A diagnosis can challenge this, forcing them to redefine who they are. Imagine someone who has always been the rock of the family suddenly needing assistance with daily tasks. Likewise, for those who found purpose in physical strength or activity, losing that ability can feel devastating. These changes extend beyond practical adjustments – they can shake a person's sense of self, making empathy and reassurance even more important.

When abilities decline gradually, grief unfolds over time. Every new limitation – whether difficulty walking, losing fine motor skills or struggling with communication – can feel like a small loss, chipping away at independence. This grief isn't a single event, but a continuous process of adaptation.

Adding to this challenge is the unpredictability of their condition. Treatments may cause unexpected side effects; chronic illnesses can flare up without warning and progressive diseases slowly diminish their capabilities. This uncertainty can create a sense of helplessness, amplifying emotional distress. Acknowledging this loss of control – both for them and yourself – can ease the burden. Offering small choices, even in daily decisions, can restore a sense of autonomy, while open conversations about your shared struggles can strengthen your bond.

Grief in these circumstances is rarely linear. One day, your loved one may seem to accept their situation, only to be overwhelmed by sadness or frustration the next. This emotional cycle requires ongoing patience and understanding. Creating an environment where emotions can be expressed freely – without fear of judgment – allows both of you to process feelings in a healthy way.

Supporting your loved one through this emotional journey requires time, empathy and honest communication. Seeking professional counselling or joining support groups can provide them with a space to process their emotions and connect with others who understand their struggles. At the same time, don't overlook your own emotional well-being. You are also experiencing a profound shift and acknowledging your grief can strengthen your connection.

There is no perfect way to navigate this journey. However, by approaching it with compassion, patience and openness, you can help your loved one find moments of dignity and peace amid the challenges. Together, you can move forward with resilience and hope.

How to Deal With the Emotional Cycle

Emotions after life-changing news aren't a straight line. You might feel fear one moment, grief the next and then suddenly be overwhelmed by guilt. That's normal. These feelings will come and go in cycles and it's okay to feel like you're looping through them.

Fear is natural when faced with uncertainty. You might find yourself wondering how you'll cope or what this means for the future. Fear isn't your enemy; it's your brain's way of urging you to prepare. Acknowledging fear is the first step to managing it.

Grieving isn't just for losing a loved one. You can grieve the loss of a life you planned, routines you cherished or dreams that now feel out of reach. Letting yourself mourn these things is part of the healing process.

Guilt often creeps in with thoughts like, 'Could I have done something to prevent this?' or 'I should be handling this better.' It can be heavy, but it's often tied to unrealistic expectations we set for ourselves. Be kind to yourself – you're doing your best.

It's okay to feel angry at the situation at how unfair it feels or even at yourself. Anger can be a sign that you care deeply and want things to be different. Use it as fuel to advocate for yourself or find solutions.

Acceptance doesn't mean you're over it. It means you've found a way to live with what's happened. Hope isn't about ignoring the hard stuff – it's about believing there are still good things ahead.

Emotions might feel overwhelming, but they're not permanent. Taking intentional steps to work through them can make a significant difference in how you feel and respond. Here's how you can start:

1. Name Your Feelings
The first step in managing your emotions is to name them. It might seem simple, but saying something like, 'I'm feeling scared' or 'I'm frustrated' allows you to create a bit of distance between yourself and the emotion. Naming your feelings gives them less power because it helps you see them as part of your experience rather than something that defines you. This practice can also help you understand what's triggering those emotions so you can address them in a meaningful way.

For instance, fear might come from uncertainty about the future, while frustration could be linked to feeling stuck or unsupported. Identifying these emotions is a powerful way to take control.

2. Find Healthy Outlets
Emotions are energy in motion and finding healthy ways to release that energy is key to moving through them. Writing in a journal can

be a great way to process what's on your mind and heart without judgment.

Talking to a trusted friend, family member or professional can also provide a sense of relief and perspective. Physical movement, like walking, running or even dancing, can help release tension and give you a boost of feel-good endorphins. It's not about finding the perfect outlet but rather discovering what works for you and allowing yourself to lean into it when emotions feel too heavy to bear.

3. Pause and Reflect

Sometimes, the best thing you can do is give yourself permission to pause. You don't need to have all the answers immediately or know exactly what to do next. Taking time to sit with your feelings allows you to process them at your own pace.

Reflection can happen in many forms – through meditation, quiet moments in nature or simply sitting in a comfortable space and letting your mind wander. This pause creates the space needed to gain clarity and insight, helping you approach challenges with a calmer, clearer mindset. It reminds you that it's okay to take your time and that clarity often comes when you least expect it.

By taking these steps, you're showing yourself compassion and building resilience, one small action at a time.

Navigating Uncertainty: Tackling the What-If's

The what-if's that creep into your mind can feel overwhelming and exhausting. 'What if I'm not strong enough?' or 'What if everything gets worse?' are common fears when facing uncertainty but you don't have to let them take over. By focusing on manageable actions and shifting your perspective, you can regain a sense of stability even when the future feels unclear. Here's how:

Focus on Today

One of the best ways to quiet the what-if's is to bring your attention to the present moment. Instead of worrying about everything that could go wrong, ask yourself, 'What can I do right now?' It might be something as simple as preparing a meal, taking a deep breath or jotting down your thoughts in a journal. Breaking things into small, actionable steps not only makes the future feel less overwhelming but also helps you feel productive and grounded. Remember, you don't need to have it all figured out – just take it one step at a time.

Seek Reliable Information

Uncertainty often feels bigger when we don't have enough information. By seeking out reliable, trustworthy sources, you can better understand what's happening and what to expect. Whether it's speaking to a healthcare provider, researching online or consulting with a professional in your situation, having accurate information helps you feel more in control. However, be mindful of limiting your exposure to overwhelming or conflicting information. Focus on what is directly relevant and actionable for your situation and don't hesitate to ask questions to clarify anything you don't understand.

Make Simple Plans

When uncertainty looms, it's easy to feel paralysed or unsure of what to do next. Making simple plans can transform that uncertainty into action. Start small – write down one or two goals for the day or week, even if they seem minor. For example, you might set a goal to schedule an appointment, prepare a comforting meal or take a 15-minute walk. These small wins add up, helping you build momentum and feel more in control of your situation. Over time, these manageable plans can grow into a roadmap for navigating the challenges ahead.

By focusing on what you can do today, equipping yourself with reliable information and creating small, achievable plans, you can manage the uncertainty and reduce the grip of the what-if's. You're stronger than you think and each step forward is a testament to your resilience.

Moving forward doesn't mean forgetting the challenges you've faced. It's about learning to carry those experiences while still creating space for joy and hope. Even in the hardest, darkest times, it's possible to find small moments that bring comfort and light. Here's how you can do it:

Practice Gratitude

Gratitude is a powerful way to shift your focus, even on difficult days. It's not about ignoring the hard stuff but noticing the small moments that bring a glimmer of happiness. It could be the warmth of a cup of tea in your hands, a kind word from someone who cares or a quiet moment when the world feels still. By recognising and appreciating these small joys, you remind yourself that even in the darkness, there are things worth holding onto. Gratitude doesn't erase pain but it helps balance it with positivity.

Celebrate Progress

Every step forward, no matter how small, is worth celebrating. Progress might look like getting out of bed on a tough morning, completing a simple task or finding a new routine that works for you. These achievements might seem minor but they are significant because they reflect your resilience and effort. Celebrating progress reminds you that you're moving forward and growing, even if the journey feels slow. Take time to acknowledge what you've accomplished – it's a way to honour your strength.

Build Your Circle

No one should have to navigate life's challenges alone. Building a supportive circle of people who care about you is essential. Whether it's family, friends or a community group, these connections can provide emotional support and practical help. Leaning on others doesn't mean you're weak – it's a way to share the load and remind yourself that you're not alone. Surrounding yourself with people who understand and care can make even the heaviest burdens feel a little lighter.

Ask for Help

Sometimes, the challenges you're facing can feel too big to manage on your own and that's okay. Speaking with a therapist or counsellor can provide a safe space to explore your emotions and gain tools to navigate them. Professional support can help you process what you're going through and give you strategies to find balance and strength. Reaching out for help is a courageous step towards healing and growth and it shows a commitment to your well-being.

This journey isn't about perfection – it's about showing up even when it feels messy or uncertain. You are not alone in this and every small step forward matters. Trust yourself to navigate the path ahead be kind to yourself when it feels overwhelming and remember that you are stronger than you think.

"Out of difficulties grow miracles." (Jean de La Bruyère)

Your strength and perseverance are proof of that truth and with each challenge you face you are creating your own miracle.

Take Action

Here are three actions you can take now to start processing your emotions and navigating this transition with greater clarity and strength.

- ✓ Name and acknowledge your feelings. Refer to *WORKBOOK 1: Processing Emotions* to guide your reflections.

- ✓ Find healthy ways to release and process your emotions
- ✓ Shift focus from uncertainty to small, actionable steps. Use *WORKBOOK 1: Planning Your Next Steps* to set your intentions and track your progress.

Taking these steps won't make the challenges disappear, but they will help you navigate them with more resilience, self-awareness and confidence in your ability to move forward.

WORKBOOK 1: Processing Emotions

Why Processing Emotions Matters

Processing emotions is one of the most important steps in navigating the journey after life-changing news. This workbook is designed to help you identify, understand and work through your emotions in a practical way. Taking just a few moments to reflect and write can make a big difference in how you feel.

Step 1: Name Your Feelings

Take a moment to identify what you're feeling right now. Use the prompts below to guide you. What emotion are you feeling most strongly at this moment? (e.g., fear, grief, anger, guilt, hope)

- **I feel:** _______________________________________
  - *What might be causing this emotion? (e.g., uncertainty about the future, a recent event, a conversation)*
- **The cause might be:**

  ____

  - *How does this emotion feel in your body? (e.g., tightness in your chest, heaviness in your limbs)*
- **It feels like:** _______________________________________

Step 2: Find Healthy Outlets

Now that you've named your feelings, think about how you can release or process them. Here are some ideas to consider:

- **Write:** Spend five minutes journaling about your feelings without judgment. Use the space below:
  - **Journal entry:**

    ____

    ____

- **Move:** Engage in a physical activity that feels good to you (e.g., stretching, walking, dancing).

- ○ **What activity could you try today?** ________________

  ____

- • **Connect:** Talk to someone who listens without judgment (e.g., a friend, family member, coach or therapist).
- ○ **Who could you reach out to?**

  ____

Step 3: Pause and Reflect

Sometimes, the best thing you can do is give yourself permission to pause. Use the following reflection prompts:

- • **What do you need right now?** (e.g., rest, reassurance, information, alone time, support)
- ○ I need: ________________
- • **What is one small thing you can do for yourself today?**
- ○ Today, I will

  ____

WORKBOOK 1: Planning Your Next Steps

Taking Action

Once you've started naming and processing your emotions, the next step is to make a plan. Planning doesn't have to mean solving everything all at once – it's about finding small, manageable actions that help you regain a sense of control. Use this workbook to guide you in creating practical and meaningful steps.

Step 1: Create a Plan

Take a moment to write down your thoughts and create a small action plan to address uncertainty or overwhelming emotions.

- **What is one thing you're worried about?**
  - I'm worried about:

  ____

- **What is one small step you can take to address it?**
  - My step:

  ____

- **What resources or tools do you need to take this step?**
  - I need:

  ____

- **Who can help you with this?**
  - I can ask:

  ____

Step 2: Practise Gratitude

Gratitude can help balance difficult emotions by focusing on positive moments. Reflect on the following:

- **What is one thing you're grateful for today?**
  ○ I'm grateful for:

  ____

- **What small joy did you experience today?**
  ○ A small joy was:

  ____

Step 3: Reflect and Revise

Planning is an ongoing process. It's important to revisit your plans and adjust as needed. Use this space to reflect:

- **Did your small step make a difference? Why or why not?**
  ○ Reflection:

  ____

- **What will you try next?**
  ○ Next step:

  ____

Final Thoughts

Taking action, even small steps, can make a big difference in how you feel. Use this workbook to revisit your plans and celebrate your progress along the way. Remember, it's not about perfection – it's about moving forward at your own pace.

CHAPTER 2

When Life Changes Overnight: The New Reality

Adjusting to a new reality can be one of the most challenging transitions in life. Receiving life-changing news often feels like being thrust into uncharted territory – filled with uncertainty, fear and questions about the future. However, the steps you take during the initial weeks and months can help you regain control and lay the foundation for long-term resilience.

The first weeks following a significant diagnosis or life event are critical. Research shows that individuals who take proactive steps early on often experience better long-term outcomes – both emotionally and practically.

According to a 2022 study from the Journal of Behavioural Medicine, those who establish support networks and create action plans within the first threemonths report a 35% higher quality of life and improvedcoping mechanisms compared to those who delay takingaction. (Journal of Behavioural Medicine, Impact of Long-Term Caregiving on Mental Resilience, 2022)

Additionally, let's have a look at some of the reasons why taking immediate action matters.

Reducing emotional overload is critical when faced with life-altering changes that can quickly spiral into overwhelm. Taking the time to break tasks into smaller, actionable steps helps you focus on what you can manage today instead of being paralysed by the enormity of the situation. For example, identifying one or two immediate priorities – like arranging medical consultations or contacting family members for support – can provide a much-needed sense of progress.

Facilitating better decision-making starts with acting quickly to gather the information and resources you need to make smart choices. For example, contacting specialists or community services early can help you avoid making decisions out of fear or stress. With the right information and support, it's easier to think clearly about options for treatment, care or support. Taking this step ensures your decisions reflect what matters most to you and your long-term goals.

Establishing a sense of control during uncertain times is key to finding your balance again. Even small proactive steps can help you feel more in charge. Planning your next move, like arranging a consultation or looking into financial assistance, shows that you are taking action toward solutions. This shift can replace feelings of helplessness with confidence and empowerment.

The initial sense of overwhelm is natural but addressing key aspects early can set you up for success and reduce unnecessary stress. Taking these steps is not about having all the answers immediately but about creating a stable starting point. By focusing on what you can control and acting with purpose, you establish a foundation for navigating this new chapter of life with greater confidence and clarity.

Taking Practical Steps: Creating Stability through Action

To navigate your new reality, it's essential to focus on a series of actionable steps. These will provide clarity and structure while ensuring that you prioritise what matters most in the early stages. In this section, we'll cover five key areas:

1. Sharing the news with others
2. Understanding and confirming the diagnosis
3. Creating a routine for normalcy
4. Incorporating self-care
5. Assembling your support network

Each topic addresses a crucial component of managing this transition, offering clear objectives and guidance to help you take control of your situation.

1. Sharing the News with Others

Sharing life-changing news with others can feel like a mountain to climb but it's a crucial first step in creating a support system. Communicating openly allows you to share the emotional load while beginning to forge connections that will help you on this journey.

After receiving such life-changing news, communicating with loved ones becomes a delicate yet necessary task. The way this news is shared can significantly influence the support system that will be vital in the months and years to come.

Opening up to others isn't just about relaying information – it's about lightening the mental and emotional weight you're carrying. When you speak with trusted individuals, you're inviting them to be part of your support network. This process creates a shared understanding, reduces feelings of isolation and fosters meaningful connections.

Psychologists have found that sharing challenges withclose friends or family members can lead to a significantdecrease in stress and anxiety levels. A study from the American Psychological Association in 2023, revealedthat individuals who openly discussed their difficultiesexperienced a 25% reduction in anxiety within the firstmonth.
(American Psychological Association, 2023)

How to Share Your News
Navigating these conversations thoughtfully can help you communicate effectively while protecting your emotional well-being. Here's how to approach it:

Start by involving a trusted circle. There may be certain individuals who should be included in the discussion sooner rather than later. Begin by sharing your situation with those you trust most – your partner, a close friend or a family member. These are the people who will likely form the core of your support network. Involving them early on can help in making informed decisions and sharing the emotional burden, ensuring that you have a strong foundation of support moving forward. These initial conversations can feel less daunting and provide the foundation for a broader support network.

Choosing the right moment and place to share your news is very important. You need to find a time when both you and your loved ones can give each other your full attention or space to share. Avoid telling them in a rushed or distracted way. Instead, pick a quiet private spot where you can talk openly without interruptions. I remember having this kind of talk with my best friend during a walk on the beach. The sound of the waves made it easier for me to gather my thoughts and being outside helped us both focus on the conversation.

As we walked, I realised how much it meant to share my feelings with someone I trusted. Letting someone in made me feel lighter and reminded me that I didn't have to face everything alone. The timing had to be right to give me the chance to open up, vent and be vulnerable about the situation and the fears and grief I felt with it.

Honesty and openness should guide your conversations. Being clear about the diagnosis, what it means and the next steps is essential. If there are uncertainties, it's okay to acknowledge them – being upfront about not having all the answers can foster trust. Loved ones may have questions and it's important to answer them as openly as possible, even if the answer is simply, 'I don't know.'

It's also important to be honest about your own emotions. You may not be ready to fully express how you're feeling and that's okay. If you need time to process the news yourself before sharing your emotions with others, don't hesitate to ask for that time. Let your loved ones know that while you may not be ready to discuss your feelings in depth right away you will do so when you feel more prepared.

Preparing for varied reactions can help you manage your expectations. Just as you have experienced a whirlwind of emotions those close to you will likely respond in different ways. Some may be shocked; others may cry and some may try to offer solutions or minimise the situation in an effort to be comforting. It's crucial to allow them their reactions – even if they are not what you expected. Encouraging open dialogue from the outset creating an environment where everyone feels heard and supported can make a significant difference as you all navigate this new reality together.

Lastly, setting clear boundaries is essential to protect your emotional well-being. Decide beforehand how much you want to share and communicate this upfront. If there are aspects of your situation, you'd prefer to keep private make that clear without guilt or apology.

What if someone reacts negatively?
It's natural to feel hurt but try to remember that their reaction may stem from their own fears or discomfort. Give them time and revisit the conversation later if necessary.

What if I'm not ready to share?
It's okay to wait until you feel prepared. Writing your thoughts in a journal can help you clarify what you want to say and how to say it.

Refer to the workbook at the end of this chapter to actively prepare: *WORKBOOK 2: Preparing to Share Your News*

2. Understanding and Confirming the Diagnosis
As the initial shock begins to ease, it's natural to feel overwhelmed by a diagnosis. This moment can feel daunting but as emotions settle, taking small, practical steps can bring a sense of control. By focusing on what can be managed, you create a foundation to move forward with confidence.

Understanding the diagnosis is the first step but it takes time. Give yourself space to process before diving into research. When ready, gather information and prepare questions for your healthcare professional. Knowledge empowers you and helps you feel more in control. Seeking a second opinion, especially for complex diagnoses, can provide reassurance or new options. When my mum was diagnosed with cervical cancer, consulting other specialists opened doors to advanced treatments and gave us a clearer path forward.

If researching online, rely on trusted organisations to avoid misinformation. Having accurate information helps you make informed decisions. It's also helpful to organise key documents, such as medical records and test results, in one secure place. A simple system – whether a notebook or digital file – can make appointments, recommendations and questions easier to track.

Once you have clarity, work with your healthcare team to create a care plan. Consider both immediate steps, such as tests or treatments and longer-term support needs. If you are the primary caregiver, think about how this role fits into your life. Adjusting work hours, modifying commitments or seeking external support can ease the load and protect your well-being.

Above all, remember – you don't have to navigate this alone. With the right support, step by step, you'll find a way forward.

3. Create a Routine for Normalcy

Establishing a routine can provide structure during uncertain times. It is crucial to create an initial plan that considers the challenges ahead, such as long days at hospital visits, treatments or travelling to different facilities. Planning for enough sleep, eating nutritious meals and ensuring pets or other responsibilities are looked after can make the first few weeks and months run more smoothly.

Asking for help from others can also ease the load – having a friend walk the dog, prepare a dish to reheat for dinner or pick up groceries can make a huge difference. These small acts of support can provide peace of mind and allow you to be fully present with your loved one during this vulnerable, fragile and emotional time.

Even small actions, such as planning mealtimes, setting aside moments for relaxation or scheduling light exercise, can create a sense of normality. Routines not only help you stay grounded but also ensure you make time to care for yourself.

Refer to the workbook at the end of this chapter to actively plan:
WORKBOOK 2: Creating a Routine for Normalcy

4. Incorporating Self Care

This naturally brings us to the importance of your own self-care. Amid all the planning and adjustments, it's crucial not to neglect your own well-being.

I once heard a caregiver say, 'Who has an extra 10 minutes?' when a group of us were discussing morning self-care activities. At the time, I laughed and agreed. But eight months later, I had an epiphany: 10 minutes out of 24 hours is less than 1% of your entire day – precisely 0.69%.

When you think about it, that's such a small portion of time, yet it can have a big impact on your well-being. Right? Yet, its impact can be transformative. I often wish I could go back and speak with that same woman, the one who said, 'Who has 10 minutes?' I'd love to show her that self-care and mindfulness aren't luxuries, they are necessities and make us one awesome caregiver because of it.

Taking even a few minutes each day to pause, breathe and reconnect with ourselves can prevent burnout, reduce stress and restore our emotional balance. It helps us show up more fully – not only for our loved ones, but for ourselves. Mindfulness isn't about finding extra time; it's about reclaiming the time we already have, ensuring we nurture our well-being amidst the demands of caregiving. After all, when we care for ourselves, we're better equipped to care for others.

As a caregiver, your physical and mental health are just as important as the care you provide to your loved one. Caregiving can be emotionally and physically draining, often leading to burnout if self-care is overlooked. It's essential to carve out time for yourself, ensuring that you are eating well, getting enough sleep and finding moments to relax and recharge. Regular exercise, even something as simple as a daily walk, can do wonders for your mental and physical health.

If you find yourself struggling to cope, don't hesitate to seek counselling or support from a mental health professional. Talking through your challenges with someone who understands the pressures of caregiving can provide much-needed relief and perspective. Remember, maintaining your own health is essential for providing the best possible care to your loved one – if you're not well, it becomes much harder to care for someone else effectively, especially when they rely on you.

In recognition of the vital importance of caregiver well-being, I have dedicated an entire chapter of this book to self-care.

5. Assembling Your Support Network

As you start the planning stage, it's equally important to start assembling your support team. Identify who in your circle of family and friends can offer assistance, whether it's with practical help, emotional support or simply being there to listen. This might include tasks such as cooking meals, babysitting other children, providing transport to sports activities or giving you a day of respite by taking your loved one to their treatment or medical appointments.

Don't be afraid to ask for help – caregiving is not something that should be done alone. Often, those around you want to help and assist, even in the smallest of ways. For example, a neighbour might offer to pick up groceries for you or a friend might take over school runs for your children. These seemingly small acts of kindness can make a significant difference in managing the demands of caregiving, especially in the beginning when you're still trying to gain a grasp on caregiving needs, establishing routines and adjusting to the changes that affect both your loved one and the immediate family.

As you navigate the early stages of caregiving, it's also crucial to research resources and support mechanisms. This may include connecting with health programs funded by medical support systems, which can offer essential services tailored to your needs. For instance, support groups – whether in-person or online – can provide a wealth of information, shared experiences and emotional support from those who are dealing with similar diagnoses and conditions. These connections can save you valuable time by offering practical advice, insights and recommendations that might not be readily available elsewhere.

Additionally, exploring social media groups dedicated to discussing specific diagnoses or caregiving challenges can be incredibly helpful. These platforms often serve as communities where members share tips, resources and updates on the latest treatment options or coping strategies. Engaging with these groups can provide much-needed information and support as you learn to navigate this new reality.

It's also important to research medical and assistive supports that might be available to you. Your healthcare professional is often a good starting point, as they may already be aware of programs or initiatives that can provide assistance.

For example, in Australia, the *National Disability Insurance Scheme (NDIS)* is a government program that offers funding for various support services, including medical treatments, therapy and assistive technologies for people with disabilities. Understanding these resources early on can help you secure the necessary support and ensure that you're making the most of the options available to you.

As you gather information and begin to build your support network, remember that we will be exploring many of these topics in greater detail throughout the book. Each chapter will delve deeper into specific resources, support networks and other essential information, offering guidance to help you navigate this journey with as much knowledge and confidence as possible.

Take Action

Here are four actions you can take now to begin navigating this transition with confidence and stability:

- ✓ Prepare to share your news using *WORKBOOK 2: Preparing to Share Your News*
- ✓ Understand and confirm your diagnosis.
- ✓ Incorporate self-care.
- ✓ Establish a routine for stability using *WORKBOOK 2: Creating a Routine for Normalcy* to map out your personal plan.

Resources:

- **National Disability Insurance Agency (NDIA):** Provides funding and support for people under 65 living with disabilities through the NDIS. *www.ndis.gov.au*

WORKBOOK 2: Preparing to Share Your News

1. Who is in your trusted circle?

Write down the names of the people you feel most comfortable speaking to first:

____

2. What do you want to share?

Summarise the key points you want to communicate:
The situation or diagnosis:

____

What this means for you and your loved one:

____

Next steps (if known):

____

3. What boundaries do you want to set?

List any topics you'd prefer not to discuss or questions you are not ready to answer:

____

Creating the Right Environment

4. When and where will you have the conversation?

Identify a quiet, comfortable setting where you and your loved one can focus:
- Time: _______________________________________
- Place: ______________________________________

5. How will you manage different reactions?

Write one way you can respond to each of the following emotions:
- Shock: ______________________________________

- Tears: ________________ ________________________________

- Problem-solving attempts: ________________________________
  ____

Reflecting on Vulnerability and Connection

6. How will you prepare emotionally?
Write one way you can give yourself space to process your feelings:
____

7. What words will you use to express vulnerability?
Write a sentence to share how you're feeling:

I feel ________________ and I want to share this with you because
____.

WORKBOOK 2: Creating a Routine for Normalcy

1. Daily Planning:
List four daily tasks to establish consistency (e.g., meals, washing, exercise, rest):

1. ____
2. ____
3. ____
4. ____

2. Routine Planning:
Outline a weekly routine, including key responsibilities (e.g., medical appointments, self-care activities):

____

____

Support System:
Identify two or more people to help with routine tasks (e.g., grocery shopping, pet care):

1. ____
2. ____
3. ____

3. Self-Care Goals:
Write one activity you will do daily for yourself (e.g., reading, meditation, walk):

____

4. Reflection:
At the end of each day, write one thing you have accomplished:

____

Taking these steps can make the journey ahead smoother, ensuring both you and your loved one are supported through this time of change.

CHAPTER 3

Thrive With Support

Caring for a loved one can be both fulfilling and overwhelming. The responsibilities involved, whether you are supporting an ageing parent, a partner, a child with a disability or even managing your own care, requires a great deal of emotional, mental and physical effort. Many caregivers face isolation, exhaustion and burnout because they try to handle everything alone. However, caregiving doesn't have to be a solo journey.

Did you know that 54% of primary carers in Australia suffer from depression? (Carers Australia Survey, 2020)

This staggering statistic highlights the immense pressure caregivers face. This chapter aims to provide practical strategies for building robust support networks, utilising community resources and developing sustainable systems to help you navigate this journey with resilience and confidence.

Why is Building a Support Network Essential?

Reduces Emotional and Physical Strain
Support networks are crucial for caregivers and their loved ones. A strong support system provides practical assistance, emotional sustenance and much-needed respite, allowing you to recharge and avoid burnout. When you are supported, you can approach caregiving with renewed patience, energy and empathy, benefiting not only yourself but also your loved one.

Ensures Continuity of Care
Unexpected circumstances such as illness, emergencies or even the need for a short break mean that caregivers must have a plan in place. A reliable support system ensures that your loved one continues receiving quality care even when you need to step away.

Enhances Quality of Life for You and Your Loved One
A well-structured support network gives you breathing space, allowing you to focus on your well-being, personal time and maintaining your identity outside of caregiving. This not only benefits you but also improves the quality of care you provide.

What We Will Cover in This Chapter:
In this chapter, we will concentrate on creating a caregiving network that provides both practical and emotional support, allowing you to navigate caregiving with greater ease and confidence. We will cover the following topics:

- Understanding the importance of building a support network
- Defining key support figures
- Strategies for building long-term support networks
- Seeking professional guidance
- Building support networks for unforeseen circumstances
- Ways to expand your horizons with like-minded people

Understanding the Terms

Building a support network begins with understanding the roles and contributions of various individuals and professionals involved in caregiving. These terms clarify the types of support available and their distinct purposes:

- *Primary Caregivers* – Family members providing hands-on, often unpaid care.
- *Informal Support* – Friends, neighbours or community members offering voluntary help.
- *Formal Support* – Paid carers providing professional assistance with daily tasks.
- *Doctors and Specialists* – Medical professionals managing treatment and care.
- *Allied Health Professionals* – Therapists and specialists improving quality of life.
- *Caregiving Coaches* – Experts helping caregivers create systems, self-care strategies to reduce stress and create balance.
- *Plan Coordinators* – Professionals assisting with funding, services and care plans.
- *Community Resources* – Charities and programs offering practical and emotional support.

Each of these components plays a distinct role in creating a balanced, well-rounded support network. By leveraging a combination of informal and formal supports, alongside expert advice from allied health professionals and caregiving coaches, you can ensure all aspects of caregiving are addressed effectively.

1. Defining Key Support Figures

The first step in building a support network is recognising who can help. This can be challenging, especially when you're used to being independent. I know this struggle all too well. My mum and I have always been very independent women and asking for help felt uncomfortable – like we were admitting defeat or relying on charity. I vividly remember hesitating every time I thought about reaching out. It wasn't until people started offering their help that I realised how much others genuinely wanted to support us.

Friends began stepping forward and their kindness changed everything. Linda started bringing us dinner on Tuesdays and Thursdays, along with delicious cakes she baked herself. Stew offered to mow Mum's lawn whenever it was needed, saving me hours of work. On my busiest evenings, Hanna would visit Mum to keep her company, sip tea or coffee and watch her favourite TV shows together.

These small gestures of kindness eased so much of the pressure I was feeling and I began to see that allowing others to help wasn't a sign of weakness. It was an opportunity to strengthen our connections and lighten the load – especially with me still working and having my own family to care for. Juggling these responsibilities was overwhelming at times but the support of others made it manageable.

Once I experienced this shift, I learned how important it is to communicate openly. Begin by identifying the people already in your life – family members, friends, neighbours or colleagues – who may be able to offer assistance. Think about their strengths, interests and how they might contribute. Open and honest communication is crucial. Start conversations by sharing your caregiving challenges and specific ways they could help.

Refer to the workbook at the end of this chapter to actively engage and ask for help: *WORKBOOK 3: Reaching Out and Asking for Help*

In case you aren't sure how to approach the subject, here are some examples:

Example 1: I've been feeling a bit overwhelmed lately with everything going on. I was wondering if you might be able to help me out by running a few errands this week?

Wait for reply.

Could you pick up some groceries and stopping by the pharmacy? It would really take a load off my mind. I've got the list and money ready to hand over before you head out.

Example 2: You know, it's been a challenge juggling everything with caring for [loved one]. I'm finding it tough to get some time to recharge. Do you think you could spend a couple of hours with them one afternoon this week? It would give me a chance to catch up on some me time.

Example 3: I've noticed I'm struggling to stay on top of things at home while looking after [loved one]. It would be amazing if you could help me out with dinner a couple of nights this week? It would be a big help if you could cook while I do other jobs around the house and it would be nice to have your company over dinner, too.

As you can see from these examples, being specific provides the other person with a clear idea of where you're at and what task you're asking for. It allows them to understand exactly what's needed and gives them a chance to evaluate whether they can commit to helping.

Clear, direct requests increase the likelihood of follow-through, as people know precisely what's expected of them. On the other hand, vague requests like 'anything would be helpful' or 'whatever you think you can do' often lead to nothing being done, simply because life gets in the way. So, do yourself a favour and ask for a specific action or task – it makes it easier for others to step in and support you.

Refer to the workbook at the end of this chapter to actively engage and ask for help: *WORKBOOK 3: Identifying who can help with what*

2. Strategies for Building Long-Term Support Networks

Practicing Appreciation and Building Trust

Once you've established connections, it's important to nurture these relationships by showing appreciation. Small gestures can make a big difference in strengthening bonds and encouraging continued support. A simple 'thank you' goes a long way but thoughtful tokens of appreciation can leave an even greater impact.

Another example from my experience was when I was caring for my mother-in-law. She had an abundance of beautiful flowers in her garden and giving a small bunch as a token of thanks to those who helped was always a lovely gesture. It was something simple yet heartfelt that left people feeling valued and appreciated.

Appreciation is a powerful tool for building trust and deepening relationships. When people feel recognised for their efforts, they're more likely to continue offering support. Thoughtful actions such as handwritten notes, a small gift or even preparing a cup of tea for someone who stops by to help can make a big difference.

Remember, every favour is appreciated. I'm sure you already do this but it's worth emphasising how important it is to acknowledge and thank those who offer help. A simple 'thank you' goes a long way. When people feel their efforts are valued, they're more likely to want to help again in the future. Here are some little ideas:

Idea 1: After your friend helps you with errands, consider leaving a handwritten thank you note along with a small gift, such as a favourite snack, a potted plant or a scented candle. You might write, 'Thank you so much for helping me out with the errands this week. It really made a difference and I'm so grateful for your support.'

Idea 2: After your friend or family member spends time with your loved one, you could bake a cake or cook something special as a token of appreciation. When you give it to them, you might say, 'I really appreciate you taking the time to be with [loved one] this week. It gave me a much-needed break and I wanted to share this with you as a small thank you.'

Idea 3: If someone helps you with dinner or spends time cooking with you, you can show appreciation by offering to help them out in the future or doing something thoughtful in return. For example, 'Thank you so much for your help with dinner this week, it was such a relief. I'd love to return the favour; maybe I can help you out with something next week?'

These small gestures of kindness and acknowledgment foster a sense of mutual respect and understanding. They show people that their help truly matters and that they're an important part of your caregiving journey. When others feel appreciated and valued, they're more likely to offer their support again in the future. Taking the time to say thank you or to give a small token of gratitude can strengthen the bonds within your support network and encourage those around you to stay connected and involved. By showing appreciation, you're not just building trust – you're creating a community of care and support that makes all the difference in your journey.

3. Seeking Professional Guidance

Consulting with professionals is a proactive way to enhance your caregiving abilities. Leveraging the expertise of professionals such as social workers, therapists, plan coordinators and caregiving consultants/coaches can significantly enhance your caregiving experience. These experts can provide tailored guidance and help with your goals, caregiving strategies and systems that alleviate some of the stresses associated with caregiving.

Social workers, for example, can connect you with local resources and support services, while therapists offer emotional support and teach coping strategies for managing stress and anxiety.

Caregiving coaches, like me, can help you establish routines and practical skills that make daily tasks more manageable, freeing up time for self-care.

Additionally, specialists like occupational therapists can recommend environmental modifications to improve safety and comfort and nutritionists can develop meal plans to support both you and your loved one's health.

Evaluate your situation, identify your key challenges and communicate with others who may offer guidance or suggest whom you might speak to about specific problems. Don't hesitate to research your options. Having worked alongside healthcare providers, allied health professionals and coaches, I'm continually impressed by the expertise that today's coaches bring to their specialist fields. Their professional training and experience often lead to remarkable results for clients in a surprisingly short time.

While consultants and coaching present an alternative approach to traditional services, it's a new way of thinking that's worth exploring. By taking the time to research and make an informed decision, you might discover valuable resources. That said, consulting professionals and seeking advice is still the top priority for protecting your well-being.

4. Building Support Networks for Unforeseen Circumstances

Being prepared for unexpected events, such as your own illness, accidents or emergencies like hospitalisations, is essential. Having a reliable support network in place ensures continuous care for your loved one while protecting your own well-being and peace of mind.

Building and maintaining a strong network is crucial in these scenarios. Professionally, relationships with healthcare providers, social workers and caregiving consultants/coaches are invaluable. These professionals can offer guidance, coordinate services, step in and provide care when you're unavailable. For instance, one client arranged for their GP to conduct home visits, which eliminated the need for clinic appointments and reduced exposure to potential infections for their immunocompromised loved one.

Speaking of consultants and coaches, as part of *A1 Quality Care's* Caregiving Systems Program, I guide caregivers through planning for respite time – such as when you're plan to be away on a holiday and health emergencies. This involves creating a system where you know exactly what steps others need to take, what instructions to follow and who is responsible for what and who the emergency contacts are.

For example, ensuring that family or friends have access to a comprehensive care plan that outlines when and how to contact key individuals, such as therapists and doctors or emergency services, can be a lifesaver in unforeseen circumstances. Whether you manage this on your own or work with a coach, having a structured plan can make a world of difference for you, your loved one and those that need to step in.

Having detailed care instructions and specific plans in place helps ease the burden during emergencies, ensuring continuity of care to your loved one in a way that you have prepared and planned in advance, reinforcing the value of a strong support system. We will explore this topic in greater detail in a later chapter, including how to build professional support networks. These professional supports play a crucial role in keeping everything running smoothly while you're away, ensuring both you and your loved one are well looked after.

On a personal level, cultivating support from support workers, family, friends and neighbours creates a vital safety net. Discuss your caregiving responsibilities with those close to you and establish emergency plans they can follow. Having a list of trusted individuals to step in when needed and knowing what to do ensures that your loved one receives seamless care during critical times.

By planning for unforeseen circumstances, not only do you ensure consistent care for your loved one but you also safeguard your own health and well-being. This proactive approach allows you to manage crises with confidence, knowing your support networks are ready to assist whenever needed.

5. Ways to Expand Your Horizons with Likeminded People

While those closest to you are a vital part of your support network, it's also important to reach out beyond your immediate circle. Consider joining local or online caregiver support groups where you can connect with others who are in similar situations.

These groups provide a platform to share experiences, gain advice and receive emotional support from people who truly understand the challenges you face.

Join Local or Online Support Groups

Caregiver support groups, whether local or online, provide a safe space to connect with others in similar situations. These groups offer opportunities to share advice, gain insights and receive encouragement. Platforms like *Facebook*, *Instagram* and *LinkedIn* host many caregiver-focused communities, allowing you to interact with others, voice challenges and explore new opportunities at your convenience.

Attend Community Events

Participating in workshops, fairs or social gatherings is another way to meet people who might become part of your support system. Community events provide opportunities to engage with like-minded individuals and expand your network naturally.

Explore Special Interest Groups and Clubs

Joining activities that align with your hobbies or passions can help you connect with others on shared interests. This could be a local book club, a gardening group or even a walking club. There are also online groups for different interests, making it convenient to participate from the comfort of your own home.

Reconnect with Old Friends

If your social life has taken a backseat due to caregiving, reaching out to old friends or acquaintances can help rebuild connections. A simple message or call can rekindle relationships and potentially grow your support network.

Volunteer for a Cause

If time permits, volunteering for a cause you care about introduces you to people who share your values. It's a rewarding way to meet new people and feel more connected to your community.

Start Your Own Group
If you're seeking others with similar caregiving experiences, consider starting your own group. This could be a casual coffee catch-up, a walking group or even a regular meeting of caregivers in your area. Creating a space tailored to your needs ensures the group aligns with your priorities and interests.

Connect with Caregiver Organisations
Organisations like *Carers Australia* or state-based carer associations provide invaluable resources, including respite care, emotional support and access to workshops or helplines. Charities such as *Dementia Australia* and the *Cancer Council* also offer tailored services, specific to each diagnosis, providing practical advice and specialised information to support caregivers.

Access Community-Based Resources
Many charities and local organisations offer practical assistance, including transportation services, meal delivery and home modifications. These resources help alleviate daily caregiving pressures and support your loved one's well-being.

Engage with Professional Support Networks
Coaches and caregiving experts, including myself, often create private communities focused on specific support topics. These spaces provide a structured and safe environment to share advice, build confidence and develop new caregiving strategies. Whether through local in-person groups or virtual platforms like Facebook, engaging with these communities can offer diverse perspectives and encouragement tailored to your caregiving journey.

Health, Disability and Aged Care Industry Connections
The Australian Government offers programs to support caregivers across health, disability and aged care sectors. For individuals with a disability, the *National Disability Insurance Scheme (NDIS)* provides funding for necessary supports and services, likewise for

the older Australians, there is the Department of Health and Aged Care programs. We'll explore these resources in greater detail in future chapters.

Refer to the workbook at the end of this chapter to actively engage and plan: *WORKBOOK 3: Building Your Social Connections Plan.*

Common Concerns and How to Overcome Them

Sometimes, it's difficult to take the first steps toward building a support network, as hesitation and concerns can hold you back. Let's explore some common worries and how to overcome them.

'I don't know where to start in building a support network.'

Building a network can feel overwhelming but the key is to take it one step at a time. Start by reaching out to people you trust, such as family, friends or neighbours and share your situation. If you feel hesitant, consider finding a friend or trusted person to accompany you to an event, activity or caregiver circle. Sometimes, having someone by your side makes it easier to connect with others and reduces the initial anxiety.

Online groups can also be an excellent starting point. As mentioned, platforms like *Facebook* or *LinkedIn* offer safe spaces where you can connect with others who understand your challenges. You can simply observe, read posts or browse comments at your own pace – there's no pressure to engage. I've found great comfort in reading other caregivers' stories. Sometimes their experiences mirrored my own, offering reassurance and other times their struggles reminded me to feel grateful for what was going well. Even uplifting quotes or bits of good news helped me keep going.

'I don't want to burden others by asking for help.'

It's natural to feel this way, especially if you're someone who has always been independent. However, asking for help isn't a burden – it's a way to invite others into your caregiving journey and allow them to contribute meaningfully. People often want to help but don't know how, so your request gives them clarity.

If you're worried about joining a group or reaching out to others, remember that you don't have to dive in all at once. You can join a group and simply sit and observe. Whether it's an in-person gathering or an online forum, there's no obligation to participate actively until you feel ready. If the group doesn't feel like the right fit, you can always leave. The key is to give yourself permission to explore these opportunities without pressure. Over time, you may find that even small steps make a big difference in building trust and gaining support.

Take Action

Here are three actions you can take now to start building and strengthening your support network.

- ✓ Identify and reach out to potential supporters. Refer to *WORKBOOK 3: Identifying who can help with what.*
- ✓ Identify tasks others can help with, reach out and show appreciation. Refer to *WORKBOOK 3: Reaching Out and Asking for Help.*
- ✓ Join or create a caregiver support group. Refer to *WORK-BOOK 3: Building Your Social Connections Plan* to actively plan and maintain social engagement.

Taking these small but meaningful steps will help you expand your support network, reduce stress and create a more sustainable caregiving experience.

Resources:

- **Carers Australia:** Offers respite care, advocacy and a range of resources to support caregivers.
  www.carersaustralia.com.au
- **Dementia Australia:** Provides support, helplines, workshops and tailored information for caregivers managing dementia-related challenges.
  www.dementia.org.au
- **Cancer Council:** Delivers practical support, helplines and resources for families affected by cancer.
  www.cancer.org.au
- **National Disability Insurance Agency (NDIA):** Manages the *National Disability Insurance Scheme* (*NDIS*), providing funding and support for individuals under 65 with disabilities.
  www.ndis.gov.au
- **Department of Health and Aged Care:** Oversees aged care programs, including respite care and services for older Australians.
  www.health.gov.au
- **A1 Quality Care:** Offers a variety of workshops, support and services tailored specifically to caregivers
  www.a1-quality-care.com

WORKBOOK 3: Reaching Out and Asking for Help

Try Out These Support Ideas

Daily support ideas to ask others for:	
Baking cakes or treats	Running errands
Tidying up common areas	Doing laundry
Organising medication	Walking the dog
Helping with light housework	Picking up prescriptions
Preparing snacks or drinks	Assisting with meal planning
Watering plants	Sorting mail or bills
Providing transportation	Accompanying your LO to appointments
Helping with personal admin	Helping with garden care
Reading or chatting for company	Babysitting or pet sitting
Staying with loved one for the afternoon	Taking loved one for the weekend
Emotional connections and support ideas to ask others for:	
Going for a calming walk in nature	Visiting a favourite café for a chat
Attending yoga class together	Going to a park for fresh air and relaxation
Watching a movie together	Visiting a museum or gallery

Spending quiet time together at home	Going for a scenic drive
Attending a support group	Visiting a spiritual or meditative space
Sharing a meal together, either at home or out	Going to a bookstore or library
Practising meditation or relaxation exercises	Taking part in a creative class, like painting
Visiting a garden or botanical park	Going to the beach or lake for peaceful time
Listening to music/creating a playlist	Going to a local event or gathering
Engaging in a shared hobby, like crafting	Visiting a spa for a relaxation day

WORKBOOK 3: Identifying Who can Help With What

Map Your Social Connections

Objective: Identify and categorise the people in your life based on your relationship with them and the type of support they can offer. This exercise will help you understand your current support network and identify any gaps that need to be filled.

Instructions:

List the people in your life (family, friends, neighbours, colleagues, etc.)

Categorise them based on their relationship to you (e.g., family, friend, professional)

Indicate the type of support they can offer (e.g., emotional support, practical assistance, companionship, respite care)

Identify any gaps in your network where you may need additional support

Name	Relationship	Type of Support	Availability	Notes
e.g. Lisa	Sister	Companionship Respite	Weekends	Lisa has offered to help with company and taking LO for one weekend per month

Reflection:

Are there any gaps in your support network? If so, what types of support do you need to seek out?

Who might you approach to fill these gaps?

WORKBOOK 3: Building Your Social Connections Plan

Plan Social Activities

Objective: Regularly schedule social activities to maintain connections with others, ensuring you stay engaged and supported outside of your caregiving role.

Instructions:

List potential social activities you enjoy or would like to try.

Schedule these activities in your calendar, aiming for a regular frequency (e.g., weekly, monthly).

Consider activities that allow you to meet new people or reconnect with old friends.

Activity	Date/Time	Frequency	Location	Who With?	Notes

Reflection:

How do these activities contribute to your well-being?

____

____

Are there any new activities you would like to explore in the future?

____

____

CHAPTER 4

Self-Care = Strength

Resilience is not something you're born with – it's something you build, brick by brick, through life's challenges. As a caregiver, resilience becomes your lifeline. Without it, the emotional and physical toll can quickly overwhelm. This chapter delves into the ways you can cultivate resilience, not in one sweeping transformation but through small, deliberate acts of self-care that grow stronger over time. Think of resilience as a tree that withstands fierce storms because its roots run deep and its trunk is strong.

This chapter is dedicated to you, the caregiver, offering practical insights, real-life examples and strategies to ensure that you not only survive but thrive in your role. By focusing on building and maintaining your resilience, you are better prepared to continue delivering the high level of care that your loved ones need, while also sustaining your own physical, emotional and mental well-being, while you stay authentic to yourself!

Throughout the book, we'll explore various ways to practice mindfulness and self-care. You don't need to implement every suggestion at once – simply choose one or two that resonate with you and gradually incorporate them into your daily routine.

As you grow comfortable with one, you can slowly add another, allowing your mind, body and subconscious time to adapt and fully embrace these practices. It's a gentle, gradual process and I promise that over time, these activities will naturally become part of your everyday life. Trust me, I've been through this journey myself and it's absolutely worth it.

Caregiving requires stamina, emotional strength and adaptability. But without resilience, even the most dedicated caregivers can falter.

Why Building Resilience is Crucial for You:

Emotional Fortitude: Resilience helps you manage the emotional highs and lows that come with caregiving, reducing stress and burnout.

Physical Well-Being: It encourages habits that protect your physical health, enabling you to care for your loved one without sacrificing your own.

Improved Relationships: When you're resilient, you're better equipped to communicate and maintain healthy boundaries with loved ones and support workers.

Enhanced Problem-Solving: Resilient caregivers can approach challenges with a clearer mind and find creative solutions.

Self-Preservation: Most importantly, resilience ensures that you remain 'you' outside of your caregiving role, preserving your identity and mental health.

Fact: *Caregivers who consistently neglect self-care are at an increased risk of chronic conditions such as hypertension, heart disease and depression. Taking small steps to care for yourself can make a big difference in lowering these health risks and improving your overall well-being. Building resilience can help mitigate this risk by fostering healthier coping mechanisms.*
(Family Caregiver Alliance, Caregiver Health)

Understanding the Terms

When discussing resilience, self-care and emotional well-being, it's essential to define these terms for clarity and guidance:

- **Resilience:** The ability to bounce back, adapt and keep going through challenges. Built through practice, not just innate traits.
- **Self-Care:** Intentional acts that support mental, emotional and physical well-being, like rest, movement and joy.
- **Mindfulness:** Being fully present, observing thoughts without judgment, fostering relaxation and clarity.
- **Journaling:** Writing down thoughts to reflect, track progress and build emotional resilience.
- **Cognitive Behavioural Techniques (CBT):** A therapy method that helps reframe negative thoughts, promoting a more positive outlook.
- **Hypnotherapy:** A guided relaxation technique accessing the subconscious to release emotional burdens and foster healing. Learn more at *www.a1-quality-care.com/hypnotherapy*

What is Resilience and How Do We Build it?

Resilience is the ability to recover from challenges, adjust to change and keep going even when things are tough. It's not about avoiding stress or challenges but about navigating through them with a mindset that focuses on growth and recovery. Resilience combines emotional, mental and physical components, all of which work together to help you weather life's storms.

Now that we've established why resilience matters and what it is, let's explore practical methods to cultivate it. These approaches integrate evidence-based strategies, personal anecdotes and practical exercises you can incorporate into your routine. Here are five ways we will address to build resilience:

- Develop coping and emotional skills
- Protect your time and energy
- Engage in meaningful and growth-oriented activities
- Stay physically active and connected with nature
- Maintain self-identity

Let's look at each one of these in more detail.

1. Develop Coping and Emotional Skills

Developing emotional resilience starts with learning how to manage stress and challenging emotions effectively. Start by identifying what works for you. Deep breathing exercises can calm you in the moment, while problem-solving helps you tackle bigger challenges. Reflect on past experiences where you've successfully coped with difficulties – what strategies did you use and can they be applied now? This includes:

Journaling
Writing about your experiences can be a powerful way to process emotions and reflect on the experiences in your caregiving journey. It provides a space to express your fears and frustrations, celebrate successes and the moments that bring you joy.

Journaling helps you release your thoughts onto paper, clearing your mind and stopping the repetitive loop of worries that your subconscious constantly cycles through. Did you know that your subconscious often replays the same concerns over and over without you even realising it? This mental loop can strain your well-being in the background, affecting you more than you might be aware.

By getting these thoughts out of your head and onto the page, you create a sense of release and clarity, which can be incredibly freeing. The beauty of journaling is that it doesn't need to follow any structure – there's no right or wrong way to do it. You might find that simply jotting down whatever comes to mind, without worrying about grammar or coherence, is enough to bring some peace to your day.

Let's see if the journaling activity in this chapter sparks the motivation to give it a try for two weeks or so. Consider this as a personal experiment – commit to just a few minutes each day and see how it makes you feel. You might discover that this small, intentional practice becomes a cornerstone in your resilience-building toolkit, offering you a gentle way to process the ups and downs of caregiving while nurturing your own well-being.

Refer to the workbook at the end of this chapter to actively plan: *WORKBOOK 4: Daily Journaling Practice*

Cognitive Behavioural Techniques (CBT)
These techniques involve challenging and changing unhelpful thoughts. For example, reframing negative thoughts like 'I'm not doing enough' to 'I'm doing my best under challenging circumstances', practicing positive thinking can significantly enhance your emotional resilience.

In my one-on-one coaching sessions, we focus on transforming negative thoughts into positive ones, using techniques tailored specifically to your needs, goals and values. This is a powerful approach I regularly practice with my clients, helping them shift their mindset and build resilience.

Through these sessions, we work together to identify and challenge old, limiting beliefs, replacing them with empowering new perspectives that lift those constraints. Whether you're struggling with self-doubt, negative self-talk or simply looking for a way to navigate the complex emotions of caregiving, this coaching offers a personalised pathway to building a more resilient mindset. By addressing your unique challenges and reinforcing positive thinking, you can develop the mental and emotional tools needed to overcome obstacles and continue providing care with confidence and mainly self-compassion.

To practice on your own, you can extend your journaling by first releasing your emotions, then identifying negative thoughts and writing a positive counterpart beside them. Start by journaling for 5-10 minutes to get your feelings out.

Then, take a break – step outside to check the mailbox, make a cup of tea or look up at the sky and notice any birds. After this refreshing pause, return to your journal with a clearer perspective.

Review what you've written, highlight any negative thoughts and at the bottom of the page, write a positive counterpart for each one. It's a powerful way to build on your self-awareness and shift your mindset.

Here are some examples of how the negative can be turned into a positive:

Negative Thought	Turned into a Positive Thought
I'm not doing enough	I'm doing my best under challenging circumstances
I always fail at this	I'm learning and each attempt helps me improve
I can't handle this anymore	This is tough but I have the strength to get through it

Negative Thought	Turned into a Positive Thought
Everything is going wrong	Not everything is perfect but there are still things going right
I'm a terrible caregiver	I care deeply and I'm doing my best to support my loved one
I should do this on my own	It's okay to ask for help when I need it
Nobody understands what I'm going through	Some people may not understand but others do
I never get any time for myself	I can make small moments for myself and prioritise self-care
I'm not strong enough for this	I've handled hard situations before and I can find strength here, too
I'm a burden to others	Asking for help shows strength, not weakness
I always make mistakes	Mistakes are part of learning and they help me grow
I have no control over anything	Some things I can't control but I can focus on what I can change
Things will never get better	Things improve over time and I can take small steps to make it better
I'm so overwhelmed	I can break things down and tackle one step at a time
I'm too tired to keep going	Rest is important and I'll regain my energy to keep moving forward
I don't deserve help	Everyone deserves support, including me
Nothing I do makes a difference	The small things I do matter, even if the results are not immediate
I'll never be good enough	I am enough and I'm constantly growing and improving
I can't trust anyone to help me	There are trustworthy people who can support me if I reach out
I'm just not capable of this	I may not have all the answers but I'm capable of learning

Limit Negative Input

Be mindful of how much negative energy you allow into your life. It's easy for the negativity of others to rub off on you, affecting your mood, energy levels and ability to remain positive. Whether it's sad, nostalgic stories or being pulled into the struggles and problems of others, remember that you don't need to take on their emotional weight, especially if it drains your energy or leaves you feeling overwhelmed. It's important to recognise your own limits – if you can't remain positive while dealing with other people's challenges, it's perfectly okay to step back and protect your own well-being.

Instead, actively seek out uplifting and positive influences. Surround yourself with people and content that raise your energy, rather than deplete it. Positive affirmations can be a wonderful way to start your day or shift your mindset when you're feeling weighed down. I highly recommend finding affirmations that resonate with you.

Check out *YouTube* or explore other platforms for affirmation videos, positive quotes and uplifting insights. These small but powerful practices can help you maintain a high level of energy and a positive outlook, even when life gets challenging. By choosing to limit negative input and focus on positivity, you'll strengthen your emotional side.

2. Protect Your Time and Energy

Boundaries Matter

Self-care includes setting healthy boundaries and learning to say no when demands become overwhelming. It begins with understanding that it's okay to say 'no' – setting boundaries is key. It's easy to fall into the habit of saying 'yes' to every request but this can quickly lead to burnout. Remember, you don't have to do everything yourself – accepting help from others is important. Managing your time by prioritising more urgent tasks and postponing less critical ones allows you to maintain balance.

Having effective strategies and systems in place can make a world of difference. Tools like diaries, calendars, to-do lists and organised systems help you to truly sit, reflect, plan and then execute your tasks in a harmonious way. When you have the right tools, it's easier to manage your responsibilities without feeling overwhelmed.

Start small. Take baby steps towards this practice – whether it's delegating a task or saying 'no' when you're feeling overwhelmed, these actions, combined with effective systems, are essential for preserving your energy and well-being.

Avoid getting drawn into the drama triangle, where you feel the need to fix every problem. Instead, stay open to new perspectives and alternative ways of handling challenges. This approach helps protect your mental and emotional well-being, allowing you to provide care without sacrificing yourself in the process.

Boundaries are essential for protecting your time and mental health. Learn to say 'no' when you need to. For example, set specific times for caregiving tasks and carve out time for yourself. Explain these boundaries to others clearly and kindly – most will respect them when they understand your needs.

Practice Mindfulness
Practising mindfulness helps you stay present and reduces the emotional toll of caregiving. By focusing on the present moment, you can better manage stress and avoid being overwhelmed by future worries or past regrets.

One of the simplest yet most effective ways to nurture your resilience is to carve out just 10 minutes each day for yourself. Techniques like mindfulness, meditation, deep breathing exercises and progressive muscle relaxation can help calm your mind and reduce stress.

At first, practicing mindfulness and relaxation techniques may feel challenging, especially when your mind is racing and stillness seems difficult. However, these are practices like any other – the more you engage in them, the more natural and beneficial they become. It's completely normal for your mind to be busy in the beginning but with consistent practice, these techniques will gradually become easier, more enjoyable and something you look forward to each day.

When learning new techniques, it can be difficult to do them on your own without any guidance or support – just like if we handed you a bicycle and expected you to ride it without showing you where to sit, how to use the pedals or how to maintain balance. Mindfulness, meditation and breathing exercises are similar in that they require practice and instruction to master. So, be gentle with yourself and seek support if you need it.

I remember my own journey, where I tried for months on my own, struggling to find my way. Then, one day, someone showed me how to fine-tune my approach, teaching me to gently acknowledge my interrupting thoughts and say to my mind, 'I love you, thank you but I'll talk to you after this practice.'

That simple guidance made all the difference. It transformed my practice into something truly impactful and it can do the same for you.

Hypnotherapy to the Subconscious
Hypnotherapy is a gentle and nurturing way of tapping into the subconscious to help navigate grief, anger, sadness, stress and many other emotions. It allows you to let go of these feelings and live without the constant burden or being shadowed by them.

One caregiver shared how only couple of her hypnotherapy sessions helped her regain focus and emotional clarity during difficult times. For more information about hypnotherapy, visit my website at *www.a1-quality-care.com/hypnotherapy*

Mindfulness and relaxation techniques not only help you recharge and stay centred but, with discipline and persistence, practising these first thing in the morning or just before bed can quickly lead to inner peace. It takes consistency and practice but the benefits are well worth the effort.

3. Engage in Meaningful and Growth-Oriented Activities

Engaging in activities that bring you joy and fulfillment is vital for maintaining a sense of purpose. Whether it's painting, cooking or volunteering, these hobbies can act as an outlet for stress and a reminder that life extends beyond caregiving. For example, one caregiver shared how joining a local art class helped her reconnect with her creative side and provided a much-needed escape from daily challenges.

Additionally, investing in your own growth can be a heart-warming and rewarding journey. Imagine stepping into a workshop filled with people who share your experiences or taking a course that lights up your curiosity. These opportunities aren't just about learning new skills – they're about reconnecting with yourself and discovering passions you might have forgotten.

Whether it's a workshop, an online class or simply learning something new, these experiences can bring a sense of joy and accomplishment to your life. Here is a table of ideas to inspire you. Perhaps a bucket list to follow:

Creative Activities	Physical Activities	Personal Growth Activities
Painting or drawing	Walking or hiking	Journaling
Photography	Yoga or pilates	Reading self-help books
Writing (stories, poetry)	Gardening	Learning a new language
Playing a musical instrument	Swimming	Taking an online course
Knitting or crochet	Dancing	Meditation and mindfulness
DIY crafts	Cycling	Personal coaching sessions
Scrapbooking	Running or jogging	Volunteering for a cause
Woodworking	Weightlifting	Mentorship or coaching others
Model building	Martial arts	Public speaking
Metalworking	Golf	Financial planning courses
Car restoration	Rock climbing	Reading biographies
Photography	Fishing or Angling	Breathwork
Writing (stories, blogs)	Football (soccer)	Learning a new skill (e.g. coding)
Leathercraft	Archery	Volunteering in community
Model building	Mountain biking	Starting a blog or podcast

4. Stay Physically Active and Connected with Nature

Physical activity is one of the most effective ways to improve your mood and manage stress and it doesn't have to be complicated or intense. Something as simple as a daily walk around the block or in your local park can work wonders for your mental and emotional well-being. For me it is a walk on the beach.

Walking not only boosts your endorphins – those feel-good chemicals that help reduce stress – but also gives you a much-needed break from the confines of your daily routine, offering a fresh perspective on whatever challenges you may be facing.

If you have a dog, you already have a built-in walking companion and this can provide extra motivation to get outside. Dogs thrive on routine and exercise and they can be a wonderful reminder to take that daily walk. As you step outside, remember that you're not just fulfilling their needs; you're also giving yourself the gift of fresh air, movement and a mental reset. The simple act of walking allows you to clear your mind, breathe deeply and reconnect with the present moment.

Walking in a natural setting, like a park, can amplify these benefits. The sights and sounds of nature – birds chirping, leaves rustling, the feeling of the ground beneath your feet – can be incredibly soothing. This time spent outdoors can serve as a gentle form of mindfulness, where you focus on your surroundings and your breath, allowing your worries to fade into the background.

Even on days when you feel tired or overwhelmed, a short walk can make a significant difference. It doesn't require much effort but the rewards are substantial. Over time, this daily habit can become a cornerstone of your self-care routine, helping you maintain your resilience and well-being.

So, lace up your shoes, grab the leash (if you have a dog) and step outside. The fresh air, the movement and the connection with nature will leave you feeling refreshed and more equipped to handle whatever comes your way.

5. Maintain Self-Identity and Preservation

It's essential to remain your authentic self while navigating the responsibilities of caregiving. Your identity is more than your caregiving role and maintaining that sense of self is crucial for your emotional and mental well-being. Think about who you are at your core – what brings you joy, what makes you laugh and what gives you purpose beyond caregiving?

Take time to reflect on your goals and dreams. What do you want to accomplish in life? Perhaps it's returning to a hobby you've always loved, setting a new goal or simply finding moments of happiness in your daily routine. These small yet meaningful steps can help you stay grounded in your identity.

Being you and doing your own things in your personal time is okay. If you need time out – you need time out. If you need respite, a couple of days away or even a holiday, give yourself permission to do it. It is absolutely vital that you are selfish and preserve yourself to be your best self for you and your loved one. When you come back recharged, your relationship can flourish because you're full of life and energy.

Allow yourself to laugh and find happiness, even during challenging times. Laughter can be a powerful reminder of life's lighter side, offering a momentary reprieve and a chance to recharge. Surround yourself with activities, people and content that inspire and uplift you.

Preserving your self-identity isn't just about enjoying life; it's about recognising that you're a whole person with dreams, interests and a purpose that extend beyond caregiving. By staying true to yourself, you not only enrich your own life but also bring your best self to the caregiving role, creating a more balanced and fulfilling experience for both of you.

You might find yourself questioning things or feeling uncertain with thoughts like these:

'I don't have time for self-care.'
Start small. Even five minutes of deep breathing or a 10-minute walk can make a difference. You don't need hours to practise self-care – consistency matters more than duration.

'I feel guilty focusing on myself.'
Remember, caring for yourself is caring for your loved one. You can't pour from an empty cup. When you're at your best, you're able to provide better care.

'I'm too overwhelmed by my loved one's illness to focus on myself.'
Caring for someone with a chronic illness or disability can feel all-consuming but resilience allows you to continue giving care without losing yourself. Prioritising small acts of self-care, like taking a moment to breathe or seeking support, can help lighten the load.

Fact: *Studies show that caregivers of individuals with chronic illnesses often experience symptoms of depression and anxiety at nearly twice the rate of the general population. Building resilience can reduce these effects and improve both your well-being and your loved one's care.*
(Family Caregiver Alliance, Caregiver Health)

Take Action

Here are three actions you can take now to start strengthening your resilience:

- ✓ Commit to a two-week journaling practice using *WORKBOOK 4: Daily Journaling Practice*
- ✓ Reframe Negative Thoughts Using CBT Techniques using *WORKBOOK 4: Reflection of Thoughts Through Journaling*
- ✓ Build your resilience and set a Small, Meaningful Self-Care Boundary using *WORKBOOK 4: Deepening Resilience through Journaling*

These actions are small but powerful and will gradually strengthen your resilience, making caregiving more sustainable while preserving your well-being.

Resources:

- *A1 Quality Care* **Website:** Visit *www.a1-quality-care.com* for in-depth caregiver support, hypnotherapy resources and personalised coaching.
- **Mindfulness Apps:** Consider using apps like *Calm*, *Headspace* or *Insight Timer* for structured relaxation and meditation exercises.
- **Caregiver Support Groups:** Join *Caring Hearts, Mindful Lives*, a nurturing and encouraging private Facebook group for caregivers.

WORKBOOK 4: Daily Journaling Practice

The objective of this activity is designed to help you build a simple yet effective daily journaling practice over the next two weeks. By taking just a few minutes each day to reflect on your thoughts and feelings, you'll develop a valuable habit that can help process emotions, clear your mind and nurture your well-being.

Instructions

1. Commit to the practice: Set aside 5-10 minutes each day for journaling. Set a timer, if it helps. You don't need to worry about grammar or structure – just let your thoughts flow onto the page. Write in your journal for the next 14 days.

2. Focus areas: If not sure what to focus and write about, consider reflecting on the following areas:

- What went well today? (Celebrate your successes, big or small)
- What challenges did I face today? (Allow yourself to express frustrations or difficult moments)
- How did I feel? (Explore your emotions without judgment)
- What am I grateful for? (Highlight positive aspects of your day)

3. Use this page or a diary: You can use the template provided below or treat yourself to a new diary or notebook. After all, it's the perfect excuse to pick out a lovely, new journal!

4. Date: Number the days (e.g., Day 1, Day 2, Day 3) along with today's date.

5. Write: Let your mind guide the pen and start writing:

Day: _________

Date: _________

WORKBOOK 4: Reflection of Thoughts Through Journaling

Cognitive Behavioural Theory in Practice

The objective of this second step in journaling is to help you build emotional resilience by applying cognitive behavioural techniques. By reviewing your journal entries, you will identify any negative thoughts, challenge their validity and replace them with positive, empowering alternatives. This process encourages self-awareness and provides a practical way to shift your mindset from limiting beliefs and negative thoughts to positive and constructive messages.

Take a short break if you've just finished journaling. Step away for a moment – make yourself a cup of tea, check the mailbox or walk outside and take a few deep breaths while observing the sky. Give yourself this refreshing pause before moving on to the next step.

Instructions

1. Review your journaling notes and highlight any negative comments, such as, "I'm not doing enough."
2. Reflect on each negative thought and beneath it, write a more compassionate and constructive response, like, "I'm doing my best under challenging circumstances."
3. After writing the positive statements, read them aloud to yourself – once or even twice – to reinforce the shift in perspective.

____

____

____

____

____

____

WORKBOOK 4: Deepening Resilience through Journaling

The objective of this third step in the journaling process is to observe and reflect on the development of your resilience over the past 14 days. By identifying patterns in your thoughts, recognising emotional shifts and acknowledging personal growth, you will gain deeper insight into how your mindset and behaviours have evolved. This reflection allows you to celebrate progress, reinforce self-compassion and set new intentions for continued growth and resilience building.

Instructions

1. Read through the last 14 days of your journal carefully – page by page, word for word.
2. Take a break. Make yourself a cup of tea, check the mailbox and spend the next 10 minutes outside. Breathe in the fresh air, observe your surroundings and enjoy the moment. Set a timer if needed. Please don't skip this step – it's important to allow your subconscious mind to settle.
3. After your break, return to your journal and reflect on the last 14 days. Use the following questions to guide your thoughts and write down your reflections, focusing on how your resilience has developed over time.

Please note: It may take more than 14 days of journaling practice to fully gain insight into some of these questions and notice a mindset shift. Typically, progress is reflected upon after each month. You can also review after three and six months. Definitely review after 12 months, as the highlights will be profound after a year of this practice and reveal your growth through this length of time.

Activity Questions

1. Identify Thought Patterns

Do you recognise any recurring negative thoughts or themes. Are there certain triggers that keep arising?

____

____

____

2. Track Changes in Mindset

Do you notice any changes in how frequently negative thoughts occur or how easily you are able to reframe them? Has your mindset shifted in any noticeable ways?

____

____

____

3. Evaluate Emotional Growth

How have your emotional responses evolved over the past days? Have you felt more at ease, confident or resilient in handling challenges?

____

____

____

4. Assess Impact on Daily Life

How has this journaling process influenced your daily life? Are you noticing improvements in self-care, interactions with others or managing your caregiving responsibilities?

____

____

____

5. Celebrate Progress

What small or big wins or moments of progress have you experienced? How do these moments reflect your growing resilience?

---

6. Set New Intentions

Looking ahead, what new goals or areas of growth would you like to focus on? How can you continue to build on the resilience you've developed so far?

Reflection:

At the end of the two weeks, take a few moments to reflect on your journaling practice:

- How did the process feel?

- Did you notice any changes in your emotions or mindset?

- Will you continue the practice? Why or why not?

And Remember!

This is your personal experiment. There's no right or wrong way to journal – what matters is that you show up for yourself each day and allow space for your thoughts and feelings.

Give yourself the gift of time, reflection and release.

You might find that this practice becomes an essential tool for building resilience and nurturing your well-being as a caregiver.

PART 2:
THE CARE FRAMEWORK BLUEPRINT

Creating Stability, One System at a Time

This is where the foundation of caregiving takes shape. It's a hands-on, practical guide to mapping out systems that work for both you and your loved one.

Together, you'll discuss needs, identify priorities and build a care plan along with essential work instructions and tools to support caregiving. It's not just about organisation – it's about creating a rhythm that feels right, reducing stress and ensuring the best possible care.

Take a deep breath, lean in and let's start shaping a system that supports both you and your loved one with confidence and heart.

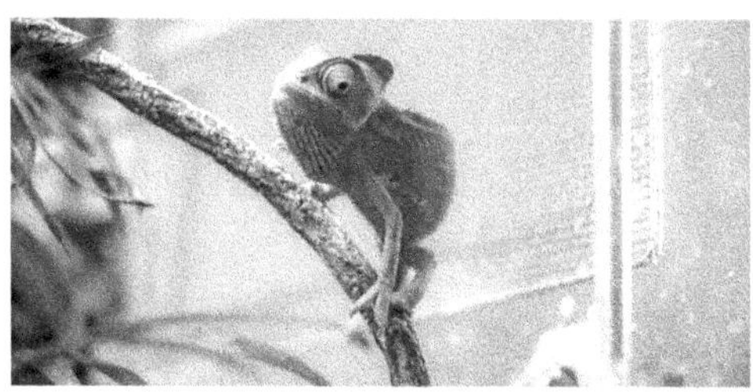

"A young chameleon watches, mimics and refines its abilities – testing colours, shifting with its surroundings and building the instincts it needs to survive. Adaptation is no longer just survival; it's a skill." (Andrea Entwistle)

CHAPTER 5

Navigating Government Supports: Making Sense of the Basics

One of the most challenging parts of caregiving is figuring out government support systems. These programs, funding options and legal considerations are constantly shifting, influenced by policies, legislation and budgets. It's easy to feel like you're falling down a rabbit hole, chasing answers that seem just out of reach. The process can be frustrating, overwhelming and at times, exhausting. But rather than getting lost in the complexity, let's focus on the essentials – the key supports available, how to access them and some personal insights that might make the journey a little easier.

Government programs exist in many countries but my knowledge and experience are deeply rooted in the Australian caregiving landscape. This chapter will explore the specific supports available here, breaking them down into practical, manageable steps.

Caring for a loved one comes with enough challenges – figuring out how to afford care, access services and navigate legal responsibilities shouldn't be an extra burden. Whether you're just beginning this journey or have been managing care for years, understanding what's available can make an enormous difference. From financial planning to *Medicare*, aged care packages and the *National Disability Insurance Scheme (NDIS)*, we'll walk through the key programs designed to help ease the load.

It's natural to worry about the financial strain of caregiving – medical expenses, home modifications, equipment and ongoing support all add up. But there are subsidies, funding programs and financial assistance options that can help, if you know where to look. Being informed about these resources means you can focus less on financial stress and more on what truly matters – caring for your loved one with confidence and peace of mind.

Many caregivers don't realise just how much support is out there. Whether it's navigating healthcare, applying for funding or accessing aged care services, the right guidance can open doors to life-changing assistance. The uncertainty of caregiving can be overwhelming, especially when unexpected needs arise but understanding what's available in advance can prevent last-minute scrambling and emotional stress.

You don't have to figure this all out alone. By breaking it down into simple, practical steps, I hope to give you the clarity and confidence to navigate these systems with ease. Let's dive in and explore what support is available, how to access it and how to make it work for you and your loved one.

In 2020, approximately 2.8 million Australians, including family members and friends, provided informal care, contributing nearly 2.2 billion hours of unpaid assistance. According to Deloitte Access Economics, the replacement value of this care was estimated at $77.9 billion. (Carers Australia, 2022)

Why Are These Important?

Caring for a loved one comes with many uncertainties and financial strain is often one of the biggest. Between medical costs, home modifications and ongoing care, the expenses can quickly add up. But support is available – you just need to know where to look. By understanding what financial assistance and subsidies exist, you can ease the burden, plan ahead and feel more secure in the choices you make for both you and your loved one.

Healthcare, insurance and *Medicare* can feel overwhelming, full of paperwork, waiting lists and confusing policies. But getting familiar with these systems can make life so much easier. Knowing how to access medical care, claim benefits and coordinate support means your loved one gets the help they need, when they need it – without added stress or unnecessary delays.

Government-funded programs like aged care packages and the *National Disability Insurance Scheme (NDIS)* can be life-changing, yet many caregivers don't realise what's available to them. These services provide home support, respite care and essential resources that can ease your daily responsibilities. By understanding how to access these supports, you can create a more balanced and sustainable caregiving journey, one where you feel empowered rather than overwhelmed.

Understanding the Terms

Let's define the key terms covered in this chapter:

- *Medicare:* Australia's universal healthcare system providing free or subsidised healthcare services, including GP visits, hospital stays and medical tests.
- *NDIS (National Disability Insurance Scheme):* A funding program supporting individuals with permanent disabilities to access necessary services, equipment and therapy.

- *Aged Care Packages:* Government-funded support services that help elderly Australians remain independent at home or transition into residential care when necessary.
- *Financial Concessions:* Rebates, discounts or subsidies for healthcare, utilities, transport and essential services to ease financial burdens on caregivers and their loved ones.
- *Power of Attorney*: A legal document granting someone the authority to make financial and medical decisions on behalf of another person if they are unable to do so.
- *Guardianship Orders*: Court-appointed responsibilities for decision-making in specific circumstances where an individual is unable to make decisions themselves.
- *Advance Care Directives*: Documents that outline a person's wishes regarding medical treatments and end-of-life care.
- *Carer Payment:* A *Centrelink*-administered financial benefit for caregivers who provide full-time support to a loved one with a disability, chronic illness or frailty due to aging.
- *Carer Allowance:* A supplementary *Centrelink* payment to assist with the costs of caring for someone who requires significant daily support.
- *Pharmaceutical Benefits Scheme (PBS):* A government program that subsidises the cost of prescription medications.
- *Hospital in the Home (HITH):* A program allowing eligible patients to receive hospital-level medical care at home, reducing hospital stays while maintaining professional healthcare support.
- *Respite Care:* Short-term care services allowing caregivers to take a break while ensuring their loved one is cared for.
- *Local Area Coordinators (LACs): NDIS* representatives who assist participants in navigating the scheme and accessing relevant services.

How to Navigate Financial and Government Supports

These supports can feel overwhelming but understanding the key areas can make the process more manageable. This chapter will break down the essentials, helping you access the right resources with confidence.

- Financial planning and legal considerations
- Navigating healthcare, insurance and *Medicare*
- Understanding aged care packages and the *National Disability Insurance Scheme*
- Financial assistance and concessions

Let's take a closer look at each of these areas.

1. Financial Planning and Legal Considerations

Managing the financial side of caregiving can feel overwhelming but with a little planning and an understanding of available resources, you can ease the pressure and create a more secure future. To help guide you through this chapter, refer to *WORKBOOK 5: Financial Planning and Legal Checklist*, which includes checklists for budgeting, financial assistance and legal planning.

Good financial planning isn't just about managing today's expenses – it's about ensuring stability for the future. Taking stock of assets, income and government support can give you a clearer picture of what's available. While financial advisers can help with long-term planning, including Power of Attorney and health directives, professionals such as local plan managers, coordinators of aged care and *NDIS* specialists can provide practical guidance on funding options, rebates and services specific to caregiving.

A great first step is to create a simple budget that includes medical expenses, equipment, home modifications and any additional support your loved one may need. Speaking with a financial planner who specialises in disability or aged care can help you identify tax deductions, rebates and strategies to make your money go further.

Many caregivers are surprised by the amount of government support available. Programs like the *National Disability Insurance Scheme (NDIS)* and Aged Care Packages can significantly reduce the financial burden, covering essential services like therapies, equipment and respite care. Taking the time to explore these options can make a real difference – not just for your loved one but for your own peace of mind.

Legal Considerations: Understanding Your Rights and Responsibilities

Planning for your loved one's future can be one of the most emotionally challenging parts of caregiving. It's not just about paperwork – it's about ensuring they will be safe, supported and cared for, even if you are no longer able to be there. Whether you are arranging short-term assistance or preparing for long-term support, having legal safeguards in place provides peace of mind and ensures continuity of care.

To help you navigate this, refer to *WORKBOOK 5: Financial Planning and Legal Checklist*, which outlines key legal steps and advocacy resources to guide you through this process.

As a caregiver, it's important to familiarise yourself with:

- **Power of Attorney** – Granting legal authority to make financial or medical decisions on behalf of your loved one if they become unable to do so. One of my clients, a devoted wife caring for her husband with dementia, struggled when financial decisions needed urgent attention. Without Power of Attorney in place, she faced delays accessing bank accounts and organising his medical care. Once it was set up, she had the reassurance that she could act on his behalf when needed.

- **Guardianship Orders** – Court-appointed responsibilities for decision-making in specific circumstances, particularly when long-term care is required. A client of mine had a son with an intellectual disability. When he turned 18, service providers could no longer discuss his care with her due to privacy laws. By securing a Guardianship Order, she was able to continue making informed decisions about his wellbeing and support services.

- **Advance Care Directives** – Documenting your loved one's wishes regarding medical treatments and end-of-life care to ensure their voice is heard, even if they cannot express it themselves. I saw the value of this firsthand with my mum. When her health declined, having an Advance Care Directive in place meant I didn't have to make difficult medical decisions under stress. Instead of second-guessing what she would have wanted, I could simply follow the plan she had carefully set out. It gave both of us peace of mind, knowing that her wishes were respected.

- **Trust Funds** – Establishing financial security for your loved one's future, ensuring their ongoing care and support needs are met even when you are no longer there to manage their affairs. A single father caring for his daughter with a disability set up a trust fund to ensure her care needs would be met long after he was gone. This provided security, knowing she would always have financial support for housing, medical needs and daily care.

Facing these decisions can feel overwhelming but you don't have to do it alone. Advocacy services are available to guide you, offer support and help you navigate legal complexities. Organisations like the *Australian Centre for Disability Law* provide advice and representation for individuals with disabilities and their caregivers, ensuring their rights are protected.

This is a difficult but necessary step in safeguarding your loved one's future. By putting these legal supports in place, you're not just planning ahead – you're giving both yourself and your loved one the reassurance that they will always have the care and security they deserve.

2. Navigating Health Care, Insurance and Medicare

Navigating healthcare systems and dealing with insurance companies can feel overwhelming but with preparation and persistence, you can make the process smoother. When you're advocating for a loved one's health, every small effort can make a big difference. Here are some practical ways to simplify and manage healthcare with more confidence and less stress.

- **Keep Detailed Records** – Having an organised folder with medical documents, specialists' recommendations, assessments and reports, medical treatment plans, service agreements and health insurance details can save time and prevent errors. It's also essential to keep key details such as your loved one's *NDIS* number *or* Aged Care Client ID and package details, as these are often required when accessing services or funding. One caregiver I know learned this the hard way – after spending hours chasing lost documents for a funding application, they started keeping a digital and physical file, making future medical appointments and approvals much easier.
- **Understand Insurance Policies** – Health insurance can be confusing but knowing exactly what's covered can prevent unexpected costs. One mother I worked with assumed

her child's therapy sessions were included in their private health insurance, only to find out too late that they weren't. Now, before engaging in any therapy, she always checks with the provider to confirm coverage, ensuring there are no surprises. It's also much easier now to compare policies online through independent comparison companies such as *Canstar* or *Compare the Market*, which can help you find the one that best suits your needs. Many of these services offer the option to speak to a real person who can walk you through different levels of cover and suggest the most appropriate private health insurance fund for your situation. Taking the time to understand your policy can save both money and stress in the long run.

- **Build Relationships with Providers** – Having a trusted team of healthcare professionals who understand your loved one's needs can make a world of difference. A family I know struggled with rotating specialists who never seemed to grasp their son's unique needs. Eventually, they found a GP and a therapy team who communicated well and worked together, creating a care plan that made life much easier. Building these relationships takes time but it ensures continuity of care and gives you reliable people to turn to in times of need.

If challenges arise, don't be afraid to reach out for help. Patient advocacy services and legal aid organisations can assist in resolving disputes, appealing denied claims and ensuring your loved one gets the care they are entitled to.

Medicare

Medicare, Australia's universal healthcare system, is a lifeline for many caregivers, providing access to essential medical services at little to no cost. Whether it's GP visits, diagnostic tests or specialist care, *Medicare* helps ensure your loved one gets the treatment they need without financial strain.

For those with ongoing medical needs, *Chronic Disease Management (CDM)* plans allow access to subsidised allied health services like physiotherapy, podiatry and occupational therapy. One caregiver shared how this program helped their father, who was too young to qualify for the aged care pension but did not meet the criteria for disability support, regain mobility after a stroke. Without this plan, accessing rehabilitation services would have been financially out of reach. Programs like these can be life-changing, providing essential therapy that improves independence and overall quality of life.

Another valuable support is *Hospital in the Home (HITH)*, which allows eligible patients to receive hospital-level care in their own homes. A dedicated wife I met was able to have her husband's IV treatments and wound care done at home, avoiding repeated hospital stays and keeping him comfortable in familiar surroundings. This option can be a game-changer for those with complex care needs, allowing them to receive essential medical care while staying close to loved ones.

For those who cannot travel easily, *Medicare* supports home visits from doctors through certain GP services, reducing the stress of getting to a clinic. One of my clients, who was immunocompromised and also faced mobility challenges, struggled with frequent medical appointments. Every trip to the clinic was not only exhausting but also increased his risk of infection. When his GP arranged regular at-home visits, it was life-changing – he could receive the care he needed without the physical strain or health risks associated with travel. These small adjustments can make a significant difference in maintaining regular medical care while ensuring safety and comfort.

Healthcare can be daunting but knowing what's available and how to access it, it can bring a sense of control and reassurance. With the right information, support and persistence, you can ensure your loved one receives the best care possible while making life a little easier for yourself as well.

3. Understanding Aged Care Packages and NDIS

Aged Care Packages

Caring for an elderly loved one comes with many questions – who do you turn to for help? What support is available? How long does the process take? Many people are unaware of where to start and this can lead to unnecessary stress and delays in accessing much-needed care. The Australian government provides Home Care Packages designed to support older Australians in maintaining their independence while ensuring they receive the necessary care to maintain their quality of life.

The first step in accessing aged care support is arranging an *Aged Care Assessment Team* (ACAT) assessment. This is a crucial part of the process, as it determines the level of care your loved one is eligible for. The wait time for an ACAT assessment can vary depending on demand but it typically takes between six weeks to several months from the initial request to receiving an approval for services. It's important to start the process early, even if your loved one doesn't need immediate support, as wait times for services after approval can also take time.

Once an assessment is completed, your loved one will be assigned a Home Care Package level based on their needs. There are four levels, ranging from basic support to high-level care. Many families are surprised to learn that finding a provider is their responsibility, as ACAT approval does not automatically connect you to services. Approved providers, such as *My Aged Care*, *Anglicare*, *Uniting* and local aged care agencies, can assist in setting up the right services tailored to your loved one's needs.

- **Home Care** – Support with daily tasks like cleaning, meal preparation and personal hygiene, ensuring your loved one can continue living comfortably at home. Many families assume they need to take on all these responsibilities themselves, not realising that help is available to ease the burden.

- **Nursing Support** – Regular visits from qualified nurses who can assist with wound care, medication management and monitoring chronic conditions. This is particularly beneficial for those who require frequent medical attention but wish to remain at home.
- **Respite Care** – Short-term care options that allow you, as the caregiver, to take a break while ensuring your loved one is still receiving quality care. Many caregivers feel guilty about needing rest but respite services are designed to prevent burnout and ensure sustainable caregiving.
- **Social Support Programs** – Activities and group outings that help older Australians maintain social connections. Many elderly individuals experience loneliness and isolation, particularly after losing a spouse or close friends. These programs encourage interaction, fostering a sense of belonging.
- **Transport Services** – Assistance with getting to medical appointments, social activities and essential errands. Many elderly individuals struggle with mobility and transport services can make the difference between maintaining independence and feeling trapped at home.

In addition to government-funded Home Care Packages, families can choose to hire independent support workers, nurses or therapists for personalised care. This can be especially helpful while waiting for approvals or if additional support is needed. Private sole traders can assist with personal care, domestic tasks, nursing, therapy, social support and transport. Platforms like *Mable* and *Careseekers* allow you to find independent professionals or you can seek recommendations through community networks.

For those who require more intensive care, residential aged care facilities provide 24-hour support in a safe and structured environment. While many families struggle with the decision to transition their loved one to a residential care facility, it can sometimes be the best option for ensuring safety and comprehensive medical support.

Navigating the Home Care Package system can be overwhelming and delays in accessing services are common. That's why it's important to seek support early and get guidance from professionals who understand the process. Aged Care navigators, social workers and case managers can assist in explaining options, completing applications and helping families make informed decisions.

The key takeaway is don't wait until a crisis to start exploring aged care support. Many families only begin looking into services after a hospitalisation or sudden health decline, which can lead to rushed decisions and extended wait times. By starting the conversation early and understanding what's available, you can ensure your loved one gets the right support at the right time – helping them maintain independence, dignity and quality of life for as long as possible.

National Disability Insurance Scheme (NDIS)
Navigating the *National Disability Insurance Scheme (NDIS)* can feel overwhelming at first but it is designed to support both you and your loved one, making daily life more manageable and ensuring they receive the right assistance to thrive. The *NDIS* provides funding across three main areas, each tailored to different needs to improve quality of life.

- **Core Support** – Helps your loved one with everyday tasks, enabling them to live as independently as possible. This may include personal care, such as dressing, bathing and meal preparation or assistance with transport to work, education or community activities. Funding can also cover essential items like continence products and assistive technology, as well as opportunities for social and recreational activities that foster connection and inclusion. Knowing that your loved one has access to these supports can help ease your worries and allow them to live with more dignity and independence.

- **Capacity Building Support** – Focuses on developing skills and independence over time. It includes assistance with managing *NDIS* plans, securing housing and accessing community programs. If employment is a goal, your loved one may receive support for job training and career development. Other services focus on improving communication, building relationships and maintaining physical and mental well-being through therapy, exercise and nutrition. If your loved one is in education, this funding can also assist with transitioning from school to further study or vocational training. These supports are designed to empower your loved one to reach their full potential.

- **Capital Support** – Covers major expenses that enhance safety, accessibility and quality of life. It includes funding for essential equipment such as wheelchairs and communication devices, as well as home or vehicle modifications to improve mobility and independence. If your loved one requires specialist housing, this funding may also assist in securing a safe and suitable living environment tailored to their needs.

While the *NDIS* is focused on your loved one, you also benefit from the right support system. Respite care can be funded through the *NDIS*, ensuring you have the chance to recharge while knowing your loved one is well looked after. Accessing these services can relieve stress and help you maintain a sustainable caregiving routine without feeling overwhelmed.

Applying for the *NDIS* funding may seem daunting, as it requires detailed medical assessments, documentation and a thorough review of your loved one's needs. Once approved, you and your loved one will collaborate with a planner to develop a personalised plan tailored to their specific goals and requirements.

A support coordinator can be invaluable, helping you navigate the system, manage the plan and connect with service providers. Many caregivers find that working with a Local Area Coordinator (LAC) also makes the process smoother. LACs are often the first point of contact for *NDIS* participants and play a key role in assisting with plan development, connecting families with local services and ensuring that support is effectively implemented.

If you're unsure where to start, the *NDIS* website offers a wealth of resources and local advocacy organisations can also provide guidance. Being proactive and well-prepared ensures your loved one receives the full range of support they are entitled to.

It's important to check eligibility criteria, as individuals who sustain an injury, disease or disability after the age of 65 may not qualify for the *NDIS*. Instead, they may need to apply for services through the *Aged Care Assessment Team* (ACAT). Knowing these distinctions early can help you plan ahead and ensure your loved one receives the right type of care and funding.

Caring for a loved one is an ever-evolving journey but with the right information and support, you can navigate the *NDIS* with confidence. Understanding available funding and services empowers you to make informed decisions, allowing your loved one to live with dignity, security and independence, while ensuring you also receive the support you need as a caregiver.

4. Financial Assistance and Concessions

As a caregiver, you may be entitled to financial support and concessions to help with the caring for a loved one can bring unexpected financial challenges but there are various forms of assistance available to help ease the burden. Financial support and concessions can provide much-needed relief for everyday expenses, ensuring that you can continue to provide quality care without unnecessary financial strain.

If your caregiving responsibilities prevent you from working, you may be eligible for Carer Payment, which is administered through *Centrelink*. This payment provides regular financial support to those providing full-time care for someone with a significant disability or medical condition. In addition, Carer Allowance and Carer Supplement offer extra financial assistance to help with ongoing costs such as medical expenses, home modifications and specialist equipment.

For caregivers of children with disabilities, the Child Disability Assistance Payment provides additional financial relief. This payment can help cover the extra costs associated with therapies, special education or mobility aids. Some of these payments are made automatically if you already receive certain caregiver allowances, so it's important to check your eligibility.

Beyond direct financial support, you may also be entitled to discounts and concessions on essential services such as electricity, public transport and healthcare. Many of these financial benefits are available through *Centrelink* and eligibility may vary depending on your location. Checking what is available in your local area can help you maximise the assistance you receive.

- **Taxi Subsidy Scheme** – Many states offer subsidised taxi fares for individuals with disabilities or mobility challenges, helping reduce transport costs for medical appointments, social outings and essential errands. A daughter caring for her elderly mother, who had limited mobility, found the Taxi Subsidy Scheme to be life-changing. With no access to a car and limited public transport options, they had been struggling to attend medical appointments. Once they secured the subsidy, her mother could comfortably travel to her specialist visits without financial stress.

- **Disability Parking Permit** – This national scheme allows individuals with mobility impairments to park in designated disability spaces, making access to facilities easier. One of my clients, who uses a walker and is very weak, struggles to walk long distances. Having a Disability Parking Permit has saved us many times, allowing us to park closer to entrances and preserve his energy for essential activities. Without it, even a simple outing to an appointment or the shops would be exhausting for him.

- **Companion Card** – This card allows caregivers to accompany their loved one to events, public transport and recreational activities for free or at a reduced cost. Most clients I have worked with have a Companion Card, which allows them to enjoy community access, events and places of interest with their support worker, while giving their caregivers a well-deserved break. It's a real life-changer for many, providing independence while ensuring they still have the assistance they need to participate fully in social activities.

- **Health Care Card** – A concession card issued through *Centrelink* that provides discounts on prescription medications, medical services and public transport. Most people who are eligible for this card experience dramatic cost savings, especially when it comes to ongoing medication and medical appointments. For those managing chronic illnesses or disabilities, the savings can make a significant difference in ensuring they can afford the care they need without financial strain.

Understanding the financial support options available can help you plan for the future and reduce the stress of caregiving costs. By taking advantage of these resources, you can ensure that both you and your loved one have access to the support needed for a better quality of life.

Taking the first step in exploring these options can feel daunting and that is totally understandable – so let's explore some of the main concerns that may arise.

'I don't have time to research all these supports.'
There are dedicated services, such as *My Aged Care* and *NDIS* Local Area Coordinators, that can help you navigate applications and eligibility without excessive effort. Seeking financial planners or community organisations can also provide guidance.

'I've applied for support before but the process is too complicated.'
Government support applications can be overwhelming but having documentation prepared and seeking assistance from advocacy groups or support workers can simplify the process.

'I don't think my loved one qualifies for financial aid.'
Many programs have eligibility tiers and even partial funding or concessions can provide financial relief. It is always worth checking with government agencies or community organisations to explore available options.

Actions to Take

Taking action is the first step in securing the right government supports for yourself and your loved one. Here are some practical steps to help you make the most of available resources:

- ✓ Gather documentation into one folder
- ✓ Seek professional advice
- ✓ Review your eligibility for programs and funding
- ✓ Create an application checklist
- ✓ Use *WORKBOOK 5: Financial Planning and Legal Checklist* to address the above

Resources:

- **My Aged Care**: *www.myagedcare.gov.au*

- **NDIS Website**: *www.ndis.gov.au*

- **Carer Gateway**: *www.carergateway.gov.au*

- **Centrelink Services**: *www.servicesaustralia.gov.au*

- **Australian Centre for Disability Law:**
  www.disabilitylaw.org.au

- **Health Insurance Comparison:** *www.canstar.com.au*

- **Compare The Market:** *www.comparethemarket.com.au*

- **Mable:** *www.mable.com.au*

- **Careseeker Australia:** *www.careseekers.com.au*

WORKBOOK 5: Financial Planning and Legal Checklist

Use this table to organise your finances effectively:

Task	✓
Identify all caregiving-related expenses, including medical costs, home modifications, equipment, professional caregiving and transport costs	
Create a monthly budget to track caregiving expenses	
Explore government-funded financial assistance programs (NDIS, Aged Care Packages, Carer Payment, DSP, statebased concessions)	
Consult a financial planner with expertise in aged care and disability to explore tax benefits and potential deductions	
Set up a dedicated caregiving fund or savings plan for future medical and support needs	

Legal Considerations Checklist

Use this table to stay prepared:

Task	✓
Establish Power of Attorney for financial and medical decisions	
Draft or update a will to reflect caregiving considerations and protect assets	
Arrange for Advance Care Directives that outline medical treatment preferences	
Understand the guardianship and administration process if long-term care planning is required	
Keep essential legal documents in a secure but accessible location	
Contact advocacy organisations (e.g., *Australian Centre for Disability Law*) for guidance on navigating legal challenges	

Accessing Financial Assistance Checklist

Use this checklist to explore available support programs:

Task	✓
Check eligibility for Carer Payment and Carer Allowance through *Centrelink*	
Apply for Health Care Cards or Pensioner Concession Cards for discounted medical services and prescription medications	
Research additional financial relief programs (Companion Card, Taxi Subsidy Scheme, state-based rebates)	
Maintain organised records of all expenses and applications to streamline the process	

CHAPTER 6

The Care Strategy: The Plan, Tools and Actions

Caregiving can often feel overwhelming, with an endless list of responsibilities to manage. From medical appointments and daily routines to emotional support and unexpected challenges, it's easy to feel stretched thin. Without a clear plan, the details can blur together, leading to stress, uncertainty and exhaustion.

This is where systems of care come in. By creating a structured approach, you can turn chaos into clarity, making life easier not just for yourself but for everyone involved – your loved one, medical professionals, support workers and even family and friends who step in to help. When well-organised, these systems help establish routines, streamline communication and ensure that essential tasks don't slip through the cracks.

At its core, a system is simply a set of interconnected steps working together toward a goal. Think of it like a recipe for baking a cake.

You need ingredients, instructions, equipment and a baker to bring everything together. If any part is missing – flour, an oven or even just following the steps correctly – the cake won't turn out as expected.

Caregiving works the same way. A well-designed system provides the structure needed to manage daily care, delegate tasks and prepare for the unexpected. Without it, things can become overwhelming, leading to burnout and mistakes. But with the right systems in place, caregiving becomes more sustainable, ensuring both you and your loved one are supported.

"For every minute spent organising, an hour is earned."
(Benjamin Franklin)

In this chapter, we'll explore how to build and implement systems of care that create stability, helping you stay organised, prepared and in control. We'll also discuss the practical tools, resources and strategies that can make caregiving smoother and more manageable.

Why Systems of Care Matter for Caregivers

Efficiency and time management for predictability help caregivers juggle responsibilities by reducing guesswork and streamlining tasks. Without a structured system, it's easy for things to slip through the cracks. Instead of relying on memory alone, setting up clear processes can help manage time more efficiently and remove unnecessary stress. Simple tools like daily care logs, digital reminders or checklists take the guesswork out of routines, ensuring everything runs smoothly.

Predictability is just as important for those receiving care. Having a structured routine provides stability, reduces anxiety and allows both the caregiver and their loved one to focus on what truly matters – quality time together rather than constantly firefighting tasks.

Consistency in care and empowerment through preparation ensure that care remains reliable even when multiple people are involved. Whether it's a family member stepping in to help, a paid support worker or a medical professional, everyone needs to be on the same page. Clear documentation of routines, medical needs and daily expectations makes handovers seamless and reduces confusion.

Instead of each person doing things differently, a structured system ensures uniform care that maintains a sense of stability for the loved one. By shifting the mental load from memory to a structured process, support workers can focus more on providing attentive and compassionate care rather than worrying about whether something has been done correctly.

Reducing energy waste for the loved one ensures that they do not have to constantly explain their needs or preferences every time a new caregiver steps in. A structured system minimises repetitive questions and ensures that support workers have access to all necessary information without requiring the loved one to guide them repeatedly.

This is particularly beneficial for individuals with disabilities or communication challenges, allowing them to conserve their energy for more meaningful interactions rather than exhausting themselves on clarifications and explanations.

Risk management and emergency readiness help support workers prepare for the unexpected by ensuring that essential information and resources are readily available. Emergencies can happen at any time and when they do, support workers need to act fast. Having an organised system in place ensures that critical information is easily accessible.

Keeping track of medical supplies prevents the risk of running out at a crucial moment. A care folder with medical records, emergency contacts and daily routines ensures that backup support workers can step in smoothly. Clear guidance for handling urgent situations – such as a fall, allergic reaction or behavioural escalation – removes uncertainty and ensures the right actions are taken quickly, reducing stress and improving outcomes.

Empowering loved ones and enhancing well-being allows those receiving care to maintain independence while feeling secure in their routines. When care instructions and preferences are documented, they don't have to spend energy repeatedly guiding different support workers through the same information.

Instead of relying on verbal instructions, a structured system ensures their care preferences and needs are clearly communicated to everyone involved. This preserves their dignity and independence while allowing caregivers to focus on the more meaningful parts of their relationship – spending quality time together without the constant burden of managing tasks.

According to the Australian Bureau of Statistics' 2022 Survey of Disability Ageing and Carers, approximately 5.5 million Australians – 21.4% of the population – are living with a disability.
(Australian Bureau of Statistics, 2022)

For these individuals, establishing structured routines is crucial as it provides comfort, stability and predictability, reducing anxiety and enhancing overall well-being. For caregivers, implementing such routines, also known as care plans, not only helps in managing responsibilities more effectively but also fosters confidence in delivering consistent high-quality care.

Understanding the Terms
Before diving into how to establish caregiving systems, it's important to clarify a few key terms:

- *Caregiving System* – A structured approach that combines routines, tools and resources to manage care efficiently, ensuring consistency and reducing caregiver stress.
- *Care Plan* – A personalised document that outlines a loved one's medical needs, daily routines, preferences and support requirements, ensuring all caregivers follow the same approach.
- *Support Network* – A combination of family, friends, professional caregivers and community resources that provide assistance and emotional support in caregiving responsibilities.
- *Work Instructions in Caregiving* – A detailed guide for specific caregiving tasks, ensuring they are completed correctly and consistently, reducing errors and maintaining high-quality care.
- *Record Keeping and Folder Setup* – A system for maintaining caregiving documents in both digital and physical formats. This includes a structured electronic filing system and a hardcopy folder that support workers and caregivers can easily access.

So, let's take a practical look at how you can create a system that provides consistency, reduces stress and allows for smoother caregiving transitions. You can create a clear path forward which can be achieved by focusing on the following steps:

1. Building a personalised care plan that works
2. Identifying what tasks require work instructions
3. Creating the care plan and supporting work instructions
4. Record keeping and folder setup

Each of these steps works together to build a strong caregiving system, just like baking the cake, allowing you to manage daily responsibilities without feeling overwhelmed. Let's explore each one in detail.

1. Building a Personalised Care That Works for You

Caring for a loved one comes with many moving parts and without a structured plan, it's easy to feel overwhelmed. A well-thought-out care plan brings clarity, keeps tasks organised and ensures consistency – so nothing important falls through the cracks. Without one, you might find yourself constantly juggling responsibilities, second-guessing what needs to be done next or feeling the weight of uncertainty, especially when multiple people are involved.

Having a care plan doesn't just help with organisation; it brings peace of mind. It allows you to manage your time better while ensuring your loved one receives the right level of care, even as their needs evolve. More importantly, it gives *you* breathing space.

When a daily routine is clearly outlined, others involved in care don't have to rely on your constant guidance and instructions. Instead of carrying everything in your head, this foundational document provides structure, reducing stress and giving you room to step back when needed.

The foundation of any strong care plan is a well-structured daily routine. Predictability and stability can make all the difference, particularly for those with medical conditions, disabilities or cognitive impairments. A steady routine helps keep essential tasks on track, making caregiving feel more manageable – and a little less overwhelming.

I would suggest using the provided *WORKBOOK 6: Creating a Structured Daily Routine and Support System* to be guided by the next section of the chapter to map it all out as explained here.

The first step in establishing a routine is to outline the essential daily activities that need to be completed. These will vary based on your loved one's needs, so consider adding specific times of the day where necessary for clarity. Here are some examples, you may want to include:

- **Morning routines**: Waking up, personal hygiene, dressing, breakfast and medications.

- **Daytime activities**: Meals, therapy or exercise, social engagement and appointments.

- **Evening routines**: Dinner, personal care, medication, relaxation and bedtime.

2. Identifying What Tasks Require Work Instructions

Not all caregiving tasks require detailed written instructions but for those that do, having clear documentation can ensure consistency and reduce confusion. Work instructions are particularly useful for tasks that involve specific steps, safety considerations or personalised preferences. There are several questions you want to ask when assessing support needs:

- Can my loved one complete this task safely on their own?
- Do they need reminders, supervision or hands-on assistance?
- If someone else had to take over my role today, would they need instructions to complete this task correctly?

By answering these questions, you can separate tasks into two categories, being either independent activities or assisted activities:

- **Independent Activities**: Tasks your loved one can complete on their own with little to no assistance.
- **Assisted Activities**: Tasks that require some form of caregiver involvement, whether through supervision, reminders or full physical assistance.

For any activity that requires support from another person, you should consider whether written instructions are necessary. If a task involves specific steps, safety considerations or a personal preference, having a clear set of instructions ensures that care remains consistent – even if different caregivers or support workers are involved. Here are some examples of when written instructions are beneficial:

- Administering medication
- Personal care routines
- Meal preparation
- Use of mobility aids
- Emergency procedures
- Cognitive functioning and non-verbal communication

Refer to the workbook at the end of this chapter to help you map out acitives that require a work instruction: *WORKBOOK 6: Creating a Structured Daily Routine and Support System*

3. Creating the Care Plan and Work Instructions

Care Plan

A well-structured care plan must serve as a practical guide, making caregiving more structured, predictable and efficient. To support you in creating a detailed and effective care plan, I have provided a comprehensive template that includes all key components. This template is designed to be used straight away, helping you document essential information in an organised manner and ensuring consistency in care.

Let's unpack each section of the provided workbook to understand what it is about and how you can fill it out to have an instant document that will guide others.

Refer to *WORKBOOK 6: Template Care Plan,* which provides a clear illustration of the Care Plan.

Personal Information contains comprehensive details about your loved one, such as medical history, personal routines, demographic data and preferences. This foundational information helps others understand your loved ones background and daily habits, ensuring care is provided in a personalised and respectful manner.

Assessment and Planning involves evaluating your loved one's physical, cognitive, emotional and social functioning. This assessment identifies areas where support is required and helps in setting realistic, measurable goals for care.

Identified needs provide a clear description of your loved one's specific care requirements, including assistance with daily activities, medical care and social engagement. This section ensures that all caregivers understand the necessary level of support.

Goals and Objectives define both short-term and long-term aspirations for your loved one's care, along with the steps required to achieve these goals. Establishing objectives helps track progress and make adjustments as needed. Here are some of my previous client's goals as an example:

- Live as independently as possible with appropriate support.
- Develop skills for managing daily tasks (e.g., cooking, cleaning, personal care).
- Use assistive technology or adaptive equipment to enhance independence.
- Establish and maintain connections with a *Men's Shed (MAS)* group or other social groups.
- Travel and go on holidays with my wife while ensuring personal support is in place.
- Stay active with a personalised exercise or mobility program.

Support Services and Interventions list the specific services and strategies required, such as home care visits, therapy sessions or mobility assistance. Including the frequency of these services and responsible providers ensures clarity in care delivery and accountability.

Emergency Procedures outline clear steps to follow in urgent situations, ensuring that all caregivers know how to respond effectively to unforeseen circumstances. Having a structured plan helps reduce stress and improve safety, for example:

- Medical emergencies: Seizure, allergic reaction, diabetic emergency
- Missing person/wandering: Preventative measures
- Falls and injuries: Minor falls, serious falls, cuts and bleeding, burns
- Fire and evacuation: Household fires, kitchen fire, smoke or gas leak
- Power outage or equipment failure: Essential medical equipment stops working, lack of heating and cooling
- Aggressive and/or distressed behaviours: Mental health crisis, triggers, self-harm

Review and Evaluate to ensure that the care plan remains relevant over time. Scheduled reviews allow you to assess its effectiveness and make necessary updates based on your loved one's evolving needs. I would suggest a period review date every six months however keep in mind as needs and goals change the care plan will need to be reviewed and updated accordingly.

From experience, there is nothing more important than keeping the care plan up to date. Unfortunately, I have often encountered situations where this has not been the case, making it significantly harder to provide the right care. An outdated care plan creates confusion for both primary caregivers and support workers, increasing the risk of mistakes, miscommunication and unmet needs. This can lead to unnecessary stress, an unhappy loved one and, in some cases, serious health and safety risks.

Work Instructions

Work instructions are essential for ensuring that specific caregiving tasks are performed <u>accurately, consistently and safely</u>. Just like following a recipe for the cake, that I have mentioned previously, each caregiving task needs to be clearly documented so that caregivers – whether family members or professional support workers – can follow the same steps without confusion.

A well-structured work instruction provides step-by-step guidance that removes uncertainty and improves the quality of care. This is especially important when multiple caregivers are involved. A complete work instruction should answer the following key questions:

1. **What** needs to be done to ensure care is properly provided?
2. **Why** is the task important for your loved one's care and well-being?
3. **Who** is responsible for carrying out the task?
4. **Where** is the task going to take place?
5. **When** should the task be performed?
6. **How** should the task be carried out, including step by step instructions and any special technique considerations?

Use the provided *WORKBOOK 6: Gathering Information for Work instructions* to prepare and gather all the information required in a work instruction. You can use this workbook to create any instructions you need, as it is simple to use and covers the essential foundations of developing work instructions. It will be especially useful in later chapters when we explore additional caregiving systems.

Basic Rules to Keep in Mind

Keeping Work Instructions Simple and Accessible

The best work instructions are clear, concise and easy to follow. They should be written in simple language, avoiding unnecessary complexity. You can also enhance instructions by incorporating:

- Illustrations or photos: Visual aids help others understand specific steps, making the instructions easier to follow.
- QR codes for instant access: Modern technology allows QR codes that link to digital work instructions. These can be placed on medical equipment, in the car or next to important areas (e.g., near a bathroom switch). Scanning the QR code by a phone instantly provides access to instructions. It makes it somewhat more esthetical however can also be a risk if support staff do not have access to a mobile phone at the time, so keep that in mind.

Ensuring Work Instructions Remain Up-to-Date

Work instructions should be reviewed regularly to ensure they remain accurate and relevant. Just as caregiving needs evolve, documented systems must be updated to reflect any changes. You should schedule regular reviews, perhaps half yearly and review the work instructions and check that:

- The instructions are still relevant to your loved one's needs.
- Any changes in medical conditions, routines or equipment are reflected.
- Have your loved one's wishes or choices changed.
- All caregivers are aware of the latest versions and updates.

Refer to *WORKBOOK 6: Template Work Instruction*, that provides illustration of the work instruction

4. Record Keeping and Folder Setup

Keeping records organised isn't just about paperwork – it's about peace of mind. A well-structured system ensures that essential documents, care plans and work instructions are easy to find when they're needed most. Whether you're a family caregiver juggling daily responsibilities or a support worker stepping in to provide care, having everything in one accessible place removes unnecessary stress and confusion.

Most documents today are prepared electronically, so having a well-organised digital filing system is essential. Files should be easy to locate, update and refer to, ensuring that everyone involved in care has access to the most current information. Equally, if you use hard copies, it's important to print the latest version of each document and store it in a structured folder or binder. This ensures that care instructions remain up to date, reducing errors and allowing for seamless continuity of care.

By keeping records in order – whether digitally or in print – you create a smoother caregiving experience, allowing you to focus on what truly matters: providing the best care with confidence and ease. Let's take a closer look at these systems and explore how to set them up effectively, ensuring they are easy to use, maintain and access when needed.

Setting Up a Hard Copy Folder/Binder
Setting up a physical folder, naming it 'Work Instructions Folder' should be stored in an easily accessible place, such as a dedicated drawer or shelf near the caregiving area. The folder should contain these:

- A printed copy of the care plan tand work instructions.
- Emergency contacts and medical details and allergies.
- Any specific guidelines on your loved one's needs and preferences.
- Shift logs or notes to track daily caregiving activities.

Creating a Digital Filing System

In addition to a physical folder, maintaining a digital version of caregiving documents improves accessibility and reduces paperwork. These documents may be for your personal use and management, with the option to provide printed copies to others as needed. If you prefer to give others direct access, you might consider sharing the electronic files instead. The choice is entirely yours, depending on your comfort level and preferences.

For an efficient electronic filing system, you may need to store the following documents:

- Scanned copies of the care plan (if created by an agency).
- Work instructions and emergency protocols designed by healthcare professionals or agencies.
- QR codes linked to work instructions, allowing caregivers to scan and access guidance instantly.
- Digital logs to track updates and changes in caregiving routines.

It is entirely up to you how you choose to store and share these documents. You may prefer to keep them on your personal laptop at home for private use or, if you want authorised caregivers to have access, you could consider using a shared cloud folder such as *Google Drive* or *Dropbox*. This ensures that important information is always available, up to date and easily accessible when needed, while also giving you control over who can view and update the files.

However, in my experience, one of the most valuable tools in caregiving is having a reliable way to track daily updates and key information. It's not just about storing documents – it's about making sure that essential details are recorded and easily accessible for those providing care. Many caregivers and support teams use electronic logbooks, spreadsheets or shared drive systems to document important events, medication changes, behavioural observations or general notes from the day. Having a structured system in place ensures smoother communication, prevents errors and ultimately makes caregiving more effective and less stressful for everyone involved.

You may have some reservations about these documents, so let's take a moment to explore them together.

'Creating a structured care plan is too time-consuming.'
While setting up your care plan requires some initial effort, it will ultimately save you valuable time and reduce stress. A well-organised system prevents last-minute scrambling, miscommunication and repeated explanations. By using templates and structured guidelines, you can efficiently document care routines and important details without feeling overwhelmed. Once in place, a care plan allows you to focus more on your loved one rather than constantly managing the details.

'My loved one's needs change frequently, so a care plan would quickly become outdated.'
Care plans are designed to be flexible and adaptable. By reviewing and updating it regularly, you ensure that the care plan evolves with your loved one's changing needs. Having a structured system allows you to modify routines, update medications or adjust support instructions without starting from scratch each time. Your care plan also serves as a key document shared with other supports, such as providers and support agencies, ensuring quality and continuity of care for your loved one.

'I already know what needs to be done, I don't need everything written down.'
While you may have your loved one's daily routines memorised, written documentation ensures continuity of care in your absence. If another caregiver, family member or support worker needs to step in, a structured plan prevents confusion and maintains consistency

in care. It also relieves the mental load of keeping track of every detail, making caregiving more manageable and sustainable. By putting clear systems in place, you reduce the risk of burnout and ensure that both you and your loved one are fully supported.

Take Action

Now that you have explored the importance of structured caregiving systems, it's time to put your knowledge into practice. Here are three simple steps to take action today:

- ✓ Use the provided workbook to structure your care plan: *WORKBOOK 6: Creating a Structured Daily Routine and Support System*
- ✓ Complete the workbook to identify the necessary work instructions based on the care plan and tasks at hand: *WORKBOOK 6: Gathering Information for Work Instructions*
- ✓ Create your filing system, both electronic and hard copy.
- ✓ Start using your new documents – and celebrate your progress!

By taking these steps, you will have your first real-life caregiving documents ready to support both yourself and your loved one with clarity and confidence.

Congratulations!

WORKBOOK 6: Creating a Structured Daily Routine and Support System

This workbook will help you put your caregiving plan into action by organising daily routines, identifying where support is needed and creating clear instructions for delegation. Follow each step to build a structured and easy-to-follow care plan.

Step 1: Map Out the Daily Care Routine

Instructions: Fill in this table with daily activities and note who is responsible for each task.

Day of the week: _______________________________

Time of Day	Times e.g. 7.30 am	List of Activities	Who Completes It? (loved one/caregiver/other support)
Morning			
Mid-Morning			
Lunchtime			
Afternoon			
Evening			
Bedtime			

Step 2: Identify Activities That Require Support

Instructions: Tick the boxes that apply and write any notes about the level of help needed:

Activity	Independent	Needs Supervision/ Reminders	Needs Full Assistance	Notes
	☐	☐	☐	
	☐	☐	☐	

Step 3: Determine Where Written Instructions Are Needed

Instruction: Write down any tasks that need written instructions and decide where these instructions will be stored for easy access:

Activity Requiring Assistance	Does It Need Written Instructions? (Yes/No)	Where Will Instructions Be Stored? (Care Folder/Digital Document/Other)	Written Instructions Completed?
	☐ Yes ☐ No		☐ Yes
	☐ Yes ☐ No		☐ Yes
	☐ Yes ☐ No		☐ Yes

Personal Information	Details
Name:	
Date of Birth:	
Address:	
Next of Kin:	
Emergency Contact(s):	

Personal Information	Details
Medical Condition(s):	
Physical/cognitive/emotional/social functioning details:	
Personal traits/interests/hobbies:	
Goals and objectives:	
Identified needs and support services interventions:	
Emergency procedures/work instruction/directives:	
Living arrangements:	
Additional notes:	

Day of the week: _______________________________

Time of Day	Times e.g. 7.30 am	List of Activities	Who Completes It? (loved one/ caregiver/ other support)	Refer to Work Instruction Name
Morning				
Mid-Morning				
Lunchtime				
Afternoon				
Evening				
Bedtime				

Note: Work Instructions listed above are additional to the Care Plan for further information and guidance.

Next review date: _______________________________

WORKBOOK 6: Gathering Information for Work Instructions

NAME OF WORK INSTRUCTION:

____

TASKS (WHAT): What is the purpose of the work instruction?

____

____

____

METHODOLOGY (WHY): Always include the rational. Providing a reason helps others better understand why this requirement needs to be followed.

____

____

____

PERSONNEL (WHO):

____

LOCATION (WHERE): Provide a specific location/s where it is going to happen.

____

____

____

TIME (WHEN): Provide specific time and duration, if applicable

____

____

____

OBJECTIVES (HOW): Detailed step-by-step instructions on how to complete the task/ activity. Use illustrations, pictures and photos to assist with instructions.

WORKBOOK 6: Work Instruction Template

Name of Loved One (optional): _______________________
Name of the Work Instruction: _______________________

Subheading – Task: 'What'
- What is the purpose of the Work Instruction?

Subheading – Methodology: 'Why'
- Always include the rational. Providing a reason helps others better understand why this requirement needs to be followed.

Subheading – Personnel: 'Who'
- Specify the person or role responsible for completing the task or name multiple individuals if the tasks requires a team effort.

Subheading – Location: 'Where'
- Provide Specific location/s where it is going to happen.

Subheading – Time: 'When'
- Provide specific time and duration, if applicable.

Subheading – Objective: 'How'
- Detailed step-by-step instructions on how to proceed with the tasks at hand:
    1. Use a numbering or bullet point formatting.
    2. There are examples of these incorporated into the document to illustrate the formatting of the document and overall clean look.
    3. A table is also another good way to represent the steps to be taken.

Time	Task	Who	How	Where	When	Other Relevant Documents

Subheading – Photos and Illustrations

Include photos and illustrations throughout the document or at the end for easy reference.

Relevant Documents

List other relevant documents related to the Work Instruction, such as:

- Checklist
- Record sheets and logs
- QR code

Date of Next Review:

CHAPTER 7

Structuring Caregiving Systems: Stay Organised and Empowered

This chapter is divided into mini-sections, numbered 7.1, 7.2 and so on, followed by a workbook for easy navigation. Each mini-section introduces a specific system, explains its purpose, outlines what we'll cover and guides you in building it for effective management. You'll also find action steps to help you implement these systems as you progress.

While we can't cover every detail in this book, it provides a strong foundation to get started, making caregiving more manageable and setting up a structured portfolio to support your journey.

SECTION 7.1: Personal Care Needs

Personal care is more than just hygiene; it is deeply connected to dignity independence and a sense of self. Every person has their own comfort levels when it comes to receiving support and for some even the smallest details make a world of difference. What may seem like a simple routine for a support worker can be an intimate and deeply personal experience for the individual receiving care.

Take John, for example. A reserved and modest man John was comfortable with his wife assisting him with personal care but when it came to support workers he had firm boundaries. He was happy to receive help with undressing and washing most of his body but preferred to remove his underwear himself maintaining a sense of control over his most private moments. While this might have seemed like a minor detail to support workers who are accustomed to providing full care for John, it was an essential aspect of his autonomy and dignity.

John's wishes were clear: this needed to be recorded in his care plan and followed with respect. For him it wasn't just about routine – it was about feeling heard understood and valued. His story highlights the importance of recognising each individual's preferences and integrating them into daily care practices. Personal care isn't just about cleanliness; it's about preserving identity fostering independence and adapting to the ever-changing needs of the person receiving support.

While personal care needs and routines have been explored throughout this chapter we now turn our focus to implementing a structured system that ensures consistency respect and safety in care. This system provides a nurturing framework for caregivers promoting confidence understanding and a deeper sense of connection between caregivers and those they support.

What This System Covers:

- Creating work instructions for personal care/grooming routines
- Maintaining dignity and independence in personal care
- Considering hygiene-related health concerns
- Creating a consistent adaptable routine

How to Set Up an Effective System:

1. **Create work instructions for personal care/grooming routines:** Develop clear step-by-step guidance for bathing, dressing and hygiene to ensure consistency in care. Use printed guides posters or QR codes for accessibility by others such as friends, family or support workers.

2. **Maintain dignity and independence in personal care:** Encourage autonomy by discussing care preferences and setting clear dos and don'ts. Regularly review and update plans to reflect evolving needs. (Refer to Chapter 5* for detailed discussions).

3. **Consider hygiene-related health concerns:** Ensure proper continence care disposal methods and infection prevention practices. Maintain a well-organised supply of hygiene products.

4. **Create a consistent adaptable routine:** Establish a structured daily care plan that can be adapted as needs change. Provide staff with accessible instructions for reference.

Action Steps:

- ✓ Develop a personalised daily personal care schedule reflecting individual preferences
- ✓ Create a structured care guide for others/new support staff with clear work instructions
- ✓ Implement a stock management system to track essential hygiene products and prevent shortages. Refer to *WORKBOOK 7.1: Personal Care System*
- ✓ Ensure reference materials such as posters checklists and QR codes are available for caregivers

*The following steps build upon the discussions covered in Chapter 5. Please refer to Chapter 5 in conjunction with this section for a more in-depth understanding of personal care discussions and considerations. Additionally, these action points are summarised in *WORKBOOK 7.1: Personal Care System* at the end of this chapter for easy reference.

WORKBOOK 7.1: Personal Care System

This checklist serves as a simple tool to track the implementation of a structured personal care system. Caregivers and family members can use it to ensure that all necessary tasks are completed and updated as needed. Simply check off completed tasks and make notes where necessary to reflect changes or improvements.

Checklist for Personal Care System Implementation:

Task	Completed (✓)
Work instructions created for grooming routines	
-	
-	
-	
Personal care preferences documented and updated regularly	
Hygiene product stock management system implemented	
Personal care routines adapted and accessible to caregivers	
Reference materials (posters checklists QR codes) prepared	

Personal Care Products Tally Checklist

A simple table like this can be laminated and placed in the bathroom to help caregivers and family members keep track of stock levels. This ensures essential items are available and restocked as needed. A simple yet effective way to maintain a tally.

Item	Current Stock	Item Used (Tick per use)	Reorder Level	Restock Date
Shampoo				
Conditioner		142		
Body Wash				
Toothpaste				
Denture Liquid				
Toilet Paper				
Mouthwash				
Hand Soap				
Deodorant				
Moisturiser				

SECTION 7.2: Mental Health, Triggers and Treating Situations

Caring for a loved one comes with emotional highs and lows and at times, it can feel like navigating a storm without a map. Mental health is at the heart of caregiving, both for you and the person you support. Recognising and addressing mental health concerns, behavioural triggers and emotional responses is not just about managing difficult moments – it's about fostering a nurturing environment where everyone feels safe, valued and understood.

Emotional and behavioural changes can appear in many forms – perhaps your loved one withdraws into silence or sudden outbursts disrupt the day. Anxiety may show up as repetitive questioning, restlessness or physical symptoms, while depression can manifest as exhaustion, disengagement or even irritability. Dementia, PTSD and other cognitive or psychological conditions add another layer of complexity, often making familiar interactions unpredictable.

Your own emotions as a caregiver are just as important. The ongoing stress of caregiving, combined with witnessing a loved one's struggles, can take a toll. Over time, unaddressed emotional strain can lead to burnout, impacting your ability to provide care and maintain your own well-being. This is why understanding mental health and triggers is key to both prevention and support.

What This System Covers:

- Recognising mental health concerns and behavioural triggers
- Managing emotional outbursts, anxiety or depression
- Preventing carer burnout through emotional awareness
- Supporting loved ones with dementia, PTSD or other conditions

- Developing a calming environment and structured support system

How to Set Up an Effective System:

1. **Identify Emotional and Environmental Triggers**
   Every person reacts differently to stressors. Observe and document patterns – does noise overstimulate your loved one? Does an unexpected change in routine cause anxiety? Even small details, like certain words or sudden physical touch, can be triggering. Keep a trigger log to note what situations escalate distress and what calms them.

2. **Create a Personalised Crisis Response Plan**
   A structured response plan helps everyone involved respond calmly during heightened moments. This includes:

   - Preferred calming techniques – such as playing soft music, deep breathing or grounding exercises
   - A retreat space – a safe area for de-escalation when emotions rise
   - Pre-written supportive phrases – gentle, reassuring responses that avoid confrontation

   Refer to the workbook at the end of this chapter to accomplish this plan: *WORKBOOK 7.2: Personalised Crisis Response Plan*, that provides a guide for Caregivers to Navigate Emotional and Behavioural Crises

3. **Implement Daily Mood Tracking and Routine Mental Health Check-Ins**
   Recognising emotional fluctuations early can help prevent crises. This can be as simple as noting mood shifts in a journal or using a traffic light system – green (calm), yellow (anxious), red (agitated). Routine check-ins create

opportunities to identify early signs of distress and intervene proactively.

Refer to *WORKBOOK 7.2: Daily Mood Tracking Log*

4. **Develop Coping Strategies**

   Coping tools are unique to each individual. Some may respond to music therapy, while others find comfort in sensory tools like weighted blankets or aromatherapy. Trial different approaches and adjust based on what works. Encouraging mindfulness exercises, gentle physical movement or even structured hobbies can help regulate emotions over time.

5. **Educate Caregivers and Staff on De-escalation Techniques**

   Whether you're a family carer or working with professional staff, consistent approaches to de-escalation are key. Training of others should cover:

   - Speaking calmly and reassuringly in moments of distress
   - Using redirection techniques to shift focus away from the trigger
   - Avoiding confrontational language and ensuring personal space

Action Steps:

- ✓ Set up a calming routine with known effective techniques
- ✓ Develop Personalised Crisis Response Plan using *WORKBOOK 7.2: Personalised Crisis Response Plan*
- ✓ Establish a support network for emotional resilience
- ✓ Implement a daily mood tracking routine using *WORKBOOK 7.2: Daily Mood Tracking Log*

WORKBOOK 7.2: Personalised Crisis Response Plan

A Guide for Caregivers to Navigate Emotional and Behavioural Crises

This workbook will help you identify triggers, create a step-by-step response plan and develop effective calming strategies for your loved one. Answer each section thoughtfully, using real-life situations to shape a personalised crisis response that fits your unique caregiving experience.

1. Identifying Triggers

Understand what leads to distress can help prevent emotional crises before they escalate:

- What common situations or events cause emotional distress or outbursts?
  (e.g., loud noises, changes in routine, overstimulation, unfamiliar people, physical discomfort)
- Are there any specific words, actions or environments that increase agitation?
- How does your loved one typically express distress? *(e.g., pacing, yelling, withdrawing, repetitive behaviours, crying)*

Notes:

____

____

2. Early Warning Signs

Recognise early signs of distress allows for intervention before escalation:

- What small signs indicate your loved one is becoming overwhelmed? *(e.g., fidgeting, breathing changes, clenched fists, avoiding eye contact)*

- Have you noticed any patterns in emotional changes? *(e.g., certain times of day, hunger, fatigue, overstimulation?)*

Notes:

____

____

3. De-escalation Strategies

What works best to prevent a crisis from worsening?

- What calming techniques have worked in the past? *(e.g., playing calming music, dimming lights, deep breathing, offering a sensory tool)*
- What language or tone of voice is most effective in soothing your loved one? *(e.g., slow speech, reassuring phrases, avoiding direct confrontation)*
- Are there any specific phrases you should avoid? *(e.g., commands that may cause frustration or resistance)*

Notes:

____

____

4. Creating a Safe Space

A retreat space can help manage distress:

- What physical space feels safest for your loved one during distress? *(e.g., a quiet room, a corner with familiar objects, an outdoor space?)*
- What comfort items or tools can be placed there? *(e.g., soft blankets, weighted items, calming scents, familiar objects)*

Notes:

____

____

5. Step-by-Step Crisis Response Plan
This section helps structure a clear plan for managing emotional outbursts or crises:

Step 1: Recognise the Early Signs
- What immediate actions should you take when you notice early distress signals?

Step 2: Minimise Triggers
- How can you remove or reduce the triggering factor? *(e.g., lowering noise, providing reassurance, adjusting the environment)*

Step 3: Apply De-escalation Strategies
- What specific calming techniques should you use first? *(e.g., speaking calmly, offering a distraction, using grounding techniques)*

Step 4: Encourage Recovery
- What post-crisis strategies can help ease emotions and regain stability? *(e.g., quiet time, favourite activities, reflection time)*

Step 5: Document and Adjust
- How will you track and review the effectiveness of your crisis response plan? *(e.g., journaling, discussing with other caregivers, adjusting approaches based on effectiveness?)*

---

6. Emergency Support and Contacts
Make a list of trusted emergency contacts for additional support when needed.

Contact Name	Relationship	Phone Number	Role in Crisis Plan

Final Notes and Review:

- ✓ Update your plan regularly based on new observations and experiences.
- ✓ Communicate the plan with any additional caregivers, family members or support staff.
- ✓ Remember to care for yourself – emotional crises can be challenging and having support for yourself is just as important.

SECTION 7.3: Physical Health and Wellness

Keeping your loved one active is essential for their well-being. Regular movement helps prevent stiffness, reduces pain and maintains mobility, supporting their independence for longer. A structured approach ensures that physical activity is safe, effective and part of their daily routine, making caregiving smoother and reducing the risk of injuries.

Physical well-being is also closely linked to emotional and mental health. When your loved one feels physically capable, they are more likely to engage in daily activities, socialise and maintain a sense of purpose. By planning ahead, you can help manage pain, prevent secondary health conditions and improve their overall quality of life.

If they are already following a treatment plan from allied health professionals, structured movement can complement their care. Maintaining mobility, flexibility and strength not only supports their health but also ensures that physical limitations do not lead to further deterioration.

What This System Covers:

- Establish a Weekly Movement Plan
- Use an Exercise Log to Track Progress and Adjust Strategies
- Incorporate Adaptive Equipment for Safety and Ease
- Collaborate with Healthcare Professionals to Adapt Exercise Routine

How to Set Up an Effective System

1. Establish a Weekly Movement Plan
Creating a structured movement plan helps maintain consistency and prevents physical decline. Set achievable weekly goals, such as gentle stretching, assisted walking or weight-bearing exercises suited

to their condition. Incorporate variety, including hydrotherapy, physiotherapy sessions or low-impact strength training. Keeping movement manageable ensures it remains a sustainable part of their routine.

2. Use an Exercise Log to Track Progress and Adjust Strategies
Tracking progress allows you to see what works and where adjustments are needed. An exercise log helps you record completed activities, pain levels and mobility changes. Reviewing these notes regularly allows you to refine movement plans and spot early signs of stiffness, weakness or discomfort before they become bigger issues.

3. Incorporate Adaptive Equipment for Safety and Ease
Using the right equipment makes movement safer and more comfortable. Adaptive tools such as walkers, standing aids and reclining chairs that assist with transitioning from sitting to standing can provide additional support. Ensuring the right aids are in place reduces strain and allows your loved one to move with greater confidence.

4. You Should Collaborate with Healthcare Professionals to Adapt Exercise Routines
Working with physiotherapists and other allied health professionals ensures that movement routines are safe and effective. Regular check-ins help tailor exercises to their current abilities, especially if medical conditions change. These professionals can also provide guidance on pain management strategies and recommend modifications to suit different needs.

Action Steps

- ✓ Create a simple weekly mobility planner with structured movement activities using *WORKBOOK 7.3: Weekly Mobility Planner*

✓ Record exercise progress, pain levels and changes in mobility using the weekly plan using *WORKBOOK 7.3: Weekly Mobility Planner*
✓ Schedule regular check-ins with a physiotherapist or treating allied health professional to adjust movement routines as needed using *WORKBOOK 7.3: Weekly Mobility Planner*

WORKBOOK 7.3: Weekly Mobility Planner

Purpose:

This planner helps caregivers track movement activities, monitor pain levels and observe changes in mobility. By consistently logging this information, you can ensure exercises are safe, effective and tailored to your loved one's needs.

Instructions:

1. Planned Activity: List the exercises or movement planned for the day.
2. Completed (Yes/No): Indicate whether the activity was completed.
3. Pain Level Before (1-10): Record your loved one's pain level before the activity.
4. Pain Level After (1-10): Record their pain level after the activity.
5. Mobility Changes Observed: Note any improvements or difficulties in movement.
6. Additional Notes: Include observations, challenges or recommendations for the next session.
7. Record the next Appointment date with the physiotherapist

Day	Planned Activity	Time	Completed (Yes/No)	Pain Level Before (1-10)	Pain Level After (1-10)
Monday					
Tuesday					
Wednesday					
Thursday					
Friday					
Saturday					
Sunday					

Mobility Changes Observed:

____

____

Additional Notes/Comments:

____

____

Next Appointment Date:

____

____

SECTION 7.4: Health and Medication Management

Managing health and medications isn't just about remembering doses – it's about creating a structured system that ensures continuity, safety and accessibility. Medications, vital signs and emergency care all play a crucial role in your loved one's well-being and having everything organised means you can provide the best care while reducing stress and uncertainty. A well-prepared health and medical system ensures that essential information is always on hand and care providers are informed, no matter the situation.

What This System Covers:

- Health and medical folder preparation
- Setup systems for tracking medications and dosages
- Create Instructions preventing medication errors
- Monitoring vital signs and long-term health concerns
- Creating an emergency response system for medical incidents
- Training other family members or support staff, ensuring compliance with prescribed treatment plans

How to Set Up an Effective System:

1. Health and Medical Folder Preparation

A well-organised health and medical folder ensures that all essential medical information is easily accessible and up to date. This folder should always accompany your loved one – whether at home, during respite care or at medical appointments – to provide continuity of care.

- Keep both a physical copy (stored securely but accessible) and a digital version (shared with trusted caregivers or stored securely online).

- Ensure that treating doctors, allied health professionals and support workers have access to relevant documents when needed. Include:
  - Full medication list, including prescribed and over-the-counter medications, dosages and schedules.
  - Medical history, treatment records and test results.
  - Allergy records and vaccination history.
  - Advanced Care Directive and emergency contacts.
  - Work instructions for caregivers on medication administration and health monitoring.
  - Daily logs and reports for tracking medication adherence and side effects.
  - Specialist treatment plans such as:
    - Diabetes management plan, including insulin dosages and blood sugar monitoring.
    - Asthma action plan, detailing medication use and response to worsening symptoms.
    - Epilepsy treatment plan, outlining seizure triggers, emergency responses and prescribed medication schedules.

Be sure to regularly review and update this folder to reflect any changes in medications, care plans or medical conditions.

2. Setup Systems for Tracking Medications and Dosages

Knowing how much support your loved one needs with medications helps prevent missed doses or accidental double dosing.

- **Determine their level of medication support:**
  - Prompting only – Reminding them to take their medication but allowing self-administration.
  - Self-administration – They take their medication independently, with minimal oversight.
  - Full assistance – A caregiver is responsible for preparing and administering medication.

- **Choose a tracking system that suits their needs:**
    - Webster packs – Pre-packaged medications by the pharmacy, ensuring correct dosage.
    - Pill organisers – Clearly labelled compartments for different times of the day.
    - Medication reminder apps or alarms – Digital alerts for scheduled doses.
    - Written medication charts – A simple checklist to tick off after each dose is taken.

Whichever system is used, it should be easy to follow and accessible to both caregivers and the person receiving care.

3. Create Instructions Preventing Medication Errors

Clear, written work instructions help ensure medications are given safely and correctly.

- Label medications clearly and store them in a designated area to prevent confusion.
- Encourage double-checking dosages before administering any medication.
- When administering medication, follow the **5W's** in logs and instructions:

    - **When** – The exact time the medication was given.
    - **Who** – The person administering or supervising the medication.
    - **What** – The name and dosage of the medication.
    - **Why** – The reason for administration, if applicable (e.g., pain relief, blood pressure control).
    - **Where** – The method of administration (e.g. orally, injection, topical application).

Write down specific instructions on medication administration, such as:

- o Medications that must be taken with food or on an empty stomach.
- o The exact times they need to be taken.
- o Any that cannot be crushed or split.
- o Side effects to watch for and when to report them. *Take the medication information pamphlet out of the packaging and place it in a dedicated section of the health and medical folder for easy reference by caregivers and medical professionals.*

This structured approach ensures that medication errors are minimised and all relevant information is properly recorded for accountability and continuity of care.

4. Monitoring Vital Signs and Long-Term Health Concerns

Regular health monitoring helps track progress, detect early warning signs and prevent complications. Identify which vital signs need tracking based on your loved one's medical conditions:

- **Blood pressure** for those with heart issues.
- **Glucose levels** for diabetics.
- **Oxygen saturation** for respiratory conditions.
- **Weight changes** for nutritional or fluid balance concerns.

Record these readings in a daily health log that can be reviewed by doctors and caregivers and ensure caregivers know what readings are within a safe range and when to seek medical advice, again this can be supported by a work instruction.

5. Creating an Emergency Response System for Medical Incidents

Emergencies can happen at any time, so having a clear **response plan** in place helps ensure a quick and effective reaction.

- Have a step-by-step emergency plan available in the health and medical folder.
- Ensure all caregivers know:
  - Who to contact first in a medical emergency.
  - The nearest hospital, pharmacy and emergency services.
  - Signs of a medication overdose, allergic reaction or sudden health decline.
- Keep emergency contact numbers clearly displayed in the home and the folder.

6. Training Other Family Members or Support Staff

Proper training ensures consistency in care and compliance with medical treatment plans. Medication administration and health monitoring should only be carried out by individuals who have been trained to do so safely and correctly.

- **Medication administration training**: Anyone responsible for giving medication must be properly trained in correct administration techniques, dosage tracking and recognising side effects. If they are **not trained, they should not administer medication.**
- **First Aid and CPR training**: At a minimum, caregivers should have Level 1 First Aid and CPR certification to respond appropriately to health deteriorations, medication reactions and accidents. This ensures they can provide immediate assistance while waiting for emergency medical support.
- **Understanding emergency procedures**: Caregivers and support workers must know:
  - How to respond to an adverse medication reaction or health emergency.
  - The signs of deteriorating health, such as unusual drowsiness, confusion or difficulty breathing.
  - When to escalate a situation by calling emergency services or a doctor.

Ongoing training and refreshers – Encourage caregivers to attend refresher courses on medication safety, health monitoring and emergency response to stay updated on best practices.

Ensuring that all caregivers and support staff are equipped with the right skills and knowledge improves safety, reduces the risk of medication errors and provides greater confidence in managing health concerns effectively.

Action Steps:

- ✓ Create and maintain a health and medical folder using *WORKBOOK 7.4: Health and Medical Folder Checklist*
- ✓ Implement a structured medication tracking system
- ✓ Ensure caregivers are trained in medication administration and emergency response
- ✓ Write clear work instructions for medication administration and emergency preparedness
- ✓ Create health monitoring log using *WORKBOOK 7.4: Simple Health Log for Vital Signs*
- ✓ Create administration of medication record using *WORKBOOK 7.4: Medication Administration Record Sheet*

WORKBOOK 7.4: Health and Medical Folder Checklist

A well-organised health and medical folder ensures all vital information is accessible to caregivers, medical professionals and support workers.

Use a sturdy binder with dividers and plastic pockets to keep documents secure, categorised and easy to update. Store a physical copy in a known location and have a digital backup if possible.

✓	Category	Items to Include
☐	Folder Setup and Organisation	✓ Sturdy binder with dividers and plastic pockets ✓ Clearly labelled sections for quick access ✓ Store in an accessible but secure location
☐	Medication Records	✓ Full medication list (prescribed and over-the-counter) with dosages and schedules ✓ Copies of prescriptions and dispensing history ✓ Medication information pamphlets for reference ✓ Work instructions for medication administration (e.g., how to administer, special requirements) ✓ Medication tracking log (for doses given, side effects and missed doses)
☐	Medical History and Treatment Plans	✓ Complete medical history, including past and current conditions ✓ Recent test results, scans and pathology reports ✓ Specialist treatment plans (e.g., Diabetes, Asthma, Epilepsy) ✓ Allergy records and vaccination history ✓ Advanced Care Directive and emergency contacts

✓	Category	Items to Include
☐	Vital Signs and Health Monitoring	✓ Daily health log for tracking blood pressure, glucose, oxygen saturation, temperature and bowel movements ✓ Work instructions for caregivers on how to monitor vital signs ✓ Emergency response instructions for worsening symptoms
☐	Emergency Preparedness	✓ Step-by-step emergency plan for medical incidents ✓ List of emergency contacts (doctors, pharmacies, hospitals, family) ✓ First aid and CPR guidelines for caregivers ✓ Emergency response plan (signs of overdose, allergic reaction, sudden decline) ✓ Keep emergency contact numbers clearly displayed
☐	Caregiver and Support Staff Information	✓ List of trained caregivers and their responsibilities ✓ Copies of caregiver training certificates (including First Aid and CPR) ✓ Communication logs for medical professional updates
☐	Miscellaneous	✓ Plastic pocket for extra notes, receipts or appointment cards ✓ Digital backup stored securely (USB, cloud storage or email)

WORKBOOK 7.4: Simple Health Log for Vital Signs

Keeping track of your loved one's vital signs can provide valuable insights into their health and well-being. Regular monitoring allows you to spot early signs of change, helping you and healthcare professionals respond quickly and effectively.

This workbook offers a simple and organised way to record vital information, ensuring clear communication and informed decision-making, especially during times of health decline.

Date	Time	Blood Pressure	Pulse (BPM)	Temperature (°C)	Blood Sugar (mmol/L)	Oxygen Saturation (%)	Bowel Movement	Symptoms/ Concerns

Instructions for Use:

- Fill in the log daily or as recommended by the treating doctor.
- Monitor trends over time and report significant changes to a healthcare professional.
- Keep this log inside the Health and Medical Folder for easy reference.

WORKBOOK 7.4: Medication Administration Record Sheet

This record sheet ensures accurate documentation of medication administration. Caregivers should fill in all sections using the 5Ws to track when and how medication was given. This form should be kept inside the Health and Medical Folder for reference and accountability.

Medication Administration Record Sheet

Date	Time (When)	Medication Name (What)	Dosage	Method (Where)	Reason (Why)	Administered by (Who)	Signature	Notes (Side Effects/ Concerns)

Instructions for Use:

- Fill in all details immediately after administering medication.
- Record exact times to ensure doses are spaced correctly.
- The 'Where' column should specify oral, injection, topical, etc.
- The 'Who' column must be signed by the caregiver/staff responsible for administration.
- Any side effects or concerns should be noted in the last column and reported if necessary.
- Keep this log inside the Health and Medical Folder for ongoing tracking and review.

SECTION 7.5: Nutrition and Dietary Needs

As a caregiver, ensuring proper nutrition is one of the most impactful ways you can support both your loved one's health and your own. Meal planning, preparation and managing dietary needs can feel overwhelming but with a structured system, you can reduce stress and promote better well-being for both of you. Without a plan in place, mealtimes can become chaotic, leading to skipped meals, poor nutrition or unsafe food practices.

By setting up a simple and effective nutrition system, you can create balance, ensuring that your loved one gets the right nutrients while maintaining a manageable routine. This includes structured meal planning, managing dietary restrictions, ensuring proper hydration, practising food safety and where possible, encouraging your loved one to participate in meal preparation.

What the System Covers:

Develop weekly meal plans with dietary adaptations:

- Use batch cooking and meal prep strategies
- Maintain a food log to track intake and changes
- Set up an effective nutrition system
- Educate other support staff on cooking instructions and safety measures
- Plan cooking activities together

How to Set Up an Effective System:

1. Develop Weekly Meal Plans with Dietary Adaptations
Planning meals ahead of time takes the guesswork out of daily cooking and ensures that your loved one's dietary needs are met. Start by creating a 7-day rotating meal plan based on their preferences, medical requirements and nutritional needs. If your

loved one has diabetes, heart concerns or difficulty swallowing, adapt meals accordingly. Consulting a dietitian or using national dietary guidelines can be a great resource.

Batch cooking and prepping ingredients in advance can save you time while ensuring consistency. Shopping lists based on your meal plan help streamline grocery trips and reduce food waste. The more organised you are, the easier it becomes to provide nutritious meals without unnecessary stress.

2. Use Batch Cooking and Meal Prep Strategies

Batch cooking can significantly reduce your daily workload while ensuring your loved one has consistent, well-balanced meals. Preparing meals in advance allows you to portion and freeze individual servings for easy reheating, making mealtimes more manageable on busy days.

Labelling and storing meals properly can help you stay organised and avoid the frustration of last-minute cooking. With a structured approach, you can save time while ensuring your loved one receives nutritious, home-cooked meals with minimal effort each day.

3. Maintain a Food Log to Track Intake and Changes

Keeping track of what your loved one eats can help you monitor their nutrition and identify any food-related issues. A simple food log can document meals, hydration levels and any reactions to certain foods, making it easier to adjust their diet if necessary.

Pay attention to changes in appetite, digestion and energy levels. Small tweaks to their diet can have a significant impact on their comfort and overall well-being. If your loved one has allergies or sensitivities, maintaining a record of their intake will help you avoid problematic foods and make informed adjustments.

4. Educate Other Support Staff on Cooking Instructions and Safety Measures

If other caregivers or family members are involved in meal preparation, it's essential to provide clear instructions on how to cook for your loved one based on their dietary needs. This includes detailing safe food handling practices, dietary restrictions, portion sizes and preparation techniques that align with your loved one's capabilities.

For example, if your loved one has difficulty swallowing, ensure that all caregivers understand texture modifications and proper meal presentation. Having written guidelines or a shared meal plan can help maintain consistency and prevent mistakes that could impact their well-being.

5. Plan Cooking Activities Together

Cooking can be a meaningful and engaging activity that fosters connection. Set aside time to plan meals together, look up recipes and create shopping lists for the week ahead. If your loved one is capable, involve them in small, manageable kitchen tasks such as washing vegetables, stirring ingredients or selecting meal options.

Having a designated meal planning night can make nutrition more enjoyable while reinforcing a structured routine. This approach not only ensures variety in meals but also empowers your loved one to have a say in what they eat, making the process more collaborative and fulfilling.

Action Steps:

- ✓ Create meal planning systems using *WORKBOOK 7.5: Meal Planning and Nutrition System Setup Checklist*
- ✓ Prepare and batch cook meals and freeze them (clearly labelled)
- ✓ Create daily food and liquid intake log using *WORKBOOK 7.5: Food and Liquid Intake Log*

WORKBOOK 7.5: Meal Planning and Nutrition System Setup

This checklist helps you set up and maintain an effective meal planning system, ensuring consistency and ease in caregiving.

✔ **Meal Plan Creation**
- ☐ Develop a 7-day meal plan tailored to dietary needs
- ☐ Include a mix of fresh, frozen and batch-cooked meals
- ☐ Create a shopping list based on the meal plan

✔ **Meal Preparation and Storage**
- ☐ Batch cook meals and portion them into labelled containers
- ☐ Store meals safely, following proper food handling guidelines
- ☐ Check use-by dates and rotate food stock appropriately

✔ **Meal Tracking and Adaptation**
- ☐ Maintain a food log to monitor intake and dietary changes
- ☐ Adjust meals based on observed reactions or changes in needs
- ☐ Ensure hydration by tracking daily fluid intake

✔ **Involvement and Support System**
- ☐ Educate support staff or family on meal preparation and safety measures
- ☐ Set up a routine for shared meal planning and grocery shopping
- ☐ Engage loved one in age/ability-appropriate cooking activities

WORKBOOK 7.5: Food and Liquid Intake Log

Instructions: Use this log to track meals, snacks and liquid intake throughout the day. This helps monitor dietary habits, hydration levels and identify any food-related reactions or necessary adjustments.

Date: ________________

Caregiver Name: ________________
Loved One's Name: ________________
Special Dietary Considerations: ________________

Meal and Snack Log

Time	Meal/Snack	Portion Size	Notes (Reaction, Enjoyment, Changes Needed)

Liquid Intake Log

Time	Beverage Type	Amount (ml)	Notes (Hydration Level, Preferences, Issues)

- **Daily Summary and Observations**

- **Overall Appetite:** (Good/Fair/Poor)

- **Hydration Level:** (Adequate/Needs Improvement)

- **Any Issues Noted:** ________________________________

- **Adjustments Needed for Tomorrow:**

  ____

Caregiver Notes:

____

____

SECTION 7.6: Medical Tools and Equipment

Having the right medical tools and equipment in place can make a significant difference in maintaining independence, comfort and overall quality of life for your loved one. From mobility aids to assistive technology, managing these tools effectively ensures they remain functional, safe and accessible when needed. A well-organised system for selecting, maintaining and training caregivers on equipment usage prevents unnecessary stress and ensures a smoother caregiving experience.

What This System Covers:

- Choosing the right medical tools and equipment
- Organising, storing and managing equipment
- Establishing a maintenance and replacement plan
- Training caregivers and loved ones

How to Set Up an Effective System:

1. Choosing the Right Medical Tools and Equipment
Selecting the right tools can feel overwhelming with so many options available but breaking it down into key considerations can make the process easier. The goal is to find equipment that enhances independence while reducing strain on both the caregiver and the loved one.

Consult with healthcare professionals. It's tempting to purchase equipment based on recommendations from other caregivers but everyone's needs are different. Speaking with an occupational therapist, physiotherapist or GP can provide a clearer picture of what's truly necessary. For example, while a standard walker might work for one person, another may require a rollator with a seat for resting.

- **Look into hire vs purchase options.** Some equipment may only be needed for a short time, such as crutches after surgery or a hospital bed for temporary recovery. Many suppliers offer rental options, which can be a cost-effective alternative. This also allows you to trial equipment before committing to a purchase.

- **Explore government programs and funding.** Many caregivers don't realise that financial assistance is available for medical equipment. If your loved one is eligible for the *National Disability Insurance Scheme (NDIS)*, Home Care Packages or other state-based programs, you may be able to receive funding for mobility aids, assistive technology and modifications to the home. Checking eligibility early can help ease financial burdens.

- **Consider second-hand or subsidised equipment.** In some cases, second-hand medical equipment can be a practical choice, especially for high-cost items like electric wheelchairs or hoists. Organisations and disability support groups sometimes offer refurbished equipment at reduced prices. Just ensure that any second-hand items meet safety standards and are in good working condition.

- **Think about day-to-day practicality.** Equipment should fit comfortably within the home environment and be easy to use. If a power wheelchair is too large to navigate through doorways or a hospital bed is difficult to adjust, it may cause more frustration than relief. Testing equipment in-store or requesting a trial period can prevent unnecessary purchases.

Example: Sarah, a full-time caregiver for her father, was initially told to purchase a manual wheelchair for short outings. However, after speaking with an occupational therapist, she realised that her father would benefit more from a lightweight, foldable transit chair that she could easily lift in and out of the car. She also discovered that she could apply for partial funding through her father's Home Care Package, significantly reducing the out-of-pocket cost.

2. Organising, Storing and Managing Equipment

Having medical equipment is one thing – ensuring it is easy to locate, access and use is another. Proper organisation prevents last-minute scrambles and ensures a safer, more efficient caregiving experience.

- **Designate a dedicated storage area.** Medical tools should have a clear and consistent storage space. Keeping oxygen tanks, mobility aids and other frequently used devices in a specific location prevents last-minute searches. If possible, store backup supplies in an easy-to-reach but out-of-the-way area to avoid clutter.

- **Label equipment and accessories.** If multiple caregivers or family members are involved, clear labelling can help avoid confusion. Items such as nebuliser masks, hearing aid batteries or blood pressure cuffs should be clearly marked to ensure the right tools are being used.

- **Store equipment safely and maintain hygiene.** Keep medical devices in a clean, dry and temperature-controlled space. Wheelchairs should be folded properly when not in use, oxygen tanks should be secured to avoid tipping and electronic devices should be kept away from moisture. High-contact equipment, such as shower chairs and CPAP masks, should be regularly disinfected following manufacturer guidelines.

Example: Jane kept her mother's medical supplies in a single cupboard but it often became cluttered. After implementing a labelled storage system with separate plastic tubs for wound care, respiratory aids and mobility support, it became much easier for both Jane and visiting carers to find what they needed.

3. Establishing a Maintenance and Replacement Plan

Regular maintenance ensures medical equipment remains functional, reducing the risk of sudden failures that could disrupt care. Having a structured system for managing repairs, servicing and replacements prevents overwhelming surprises.

- **Schedule routine inspections:** Just like a car, medical equipment requires regular check-ups. Wheelchairs should be inspected for loose bolts, electric beds for motor function and CPAP machines for filter changes. Set reminders to check each item monthly or as per the manufacturer's recommendation. Not only does this ensure safety and functionality but it also gives you, the caregiver, a structured plan for managing equipment. Avoiding last-minute surprises, such as a broken hoist when you need it most, helps keep caregiving as seamless and stress-free as possible.

- **Maintain an Equipment Register:** Keeping track of all medical tools in use can prevent confusion and ensure nothing is overlooked. An equipment register can include details such as:

    o Equipment name and purpose
    o Purchase or hire date
    o Warranty dates
    o Maintenance schedule
    o Repair history
    o Replacement or upgrade considerations
    o Funding sources (e.g., *NDIS*) having this information in one place helps caregivers stay organised and allows for easier communication with healthcare professionals or repair providers when needed.

- **Know where to go for repairs.** Identifying a reliable repair service in advance saves time when something breaks. Keep contact details for service providers handy and check if warranties or service plans cover repairs.

- **Plan for replacements or upgrades.** As your loved one's needs change, their equipment may require updates. Check funding options for replacements through *NDIS*, Home Care Packages or other government programs. Sometimes, suppliers offer trade-in deals for old equipment when upgrading to newer models.

4. Training Caregivers and Loved Ones

Having medical equipment is only beneficial if caregivers and loved ones know how to use it correctly. Proper training ensures safety and maximises the effectiveness of each tool.

- **Seek professional demonstrations.** Whenever possible, ask a healthcare professional to demonstrate how to use medical equipment. Physiotherapists or nurses can provide hands-on guidance for things like lifting aids or breathing devices.

- **Provide easy access to instructions.** Keep manuals and instructional videos readily available, either printed or saved on a shared device. This ensures that any caregiver, whether family or professional, can quickly reference the correct procedures.

- **Encourage refresher training.** Equipment use may evolve as the loved one's condition changes. Regularly reviewing training materials or attending refresher sessions helps keep skills up to date and prevents mistakes.

Action Steps:

- ✓ Check funding options by exploring *NDIS*, Home Care Packages and rentals for affordable equipment access
- ✓ Create an equipment register and log all equipment and plan/ track maintenance using *WORKBOOK 7.6: Equipment Register*
- ✓ Provide instructions and QR codes – write guides, record demos and attach QR codes for easy access

WORKBOOK 7.6: Equipment Register

Instructions for Use:

This Equipment Register helps you track and manage all medical tools and devices used in caregiving. Keeping an up-to-date log ensures smooth maintenance, timely repairs and organised usage. Follow these steps:

1. **Enter all equipment details** in the table below, including the purchase/hire date, purpose and funding source.
2. **Track maintenance schedules** to avoid unexpected breakdowns.
3. **Use the notes section** to record important updates, replacement needs or caregiver instructions.
4. **Review the register regularly** to ensure all equipment is functional and up to date.
5. **Attach QR codes** linking to instructional videos or manuals for quick reference.

Equipment Register Table

Equipment Name	Purpose/ Use	Purchase/ Hire Date	Cost of Equipment	Funding Source	Warranty Length	Warranty Expiry Date	Maintenance Schedule	Maintenance/ Repairs Contact	Repair Details and Cost	Notes
e.g. Wheelchair	Mobility assistance	12/01/2024	$2,000	NDIS	2 years	12/01/2027	Monthly check-up	ABC Mobility Repairs: 1234577890	Brake repair: $100	Needs servicing every 7 months

Tip: Print and place this register in an accessible location or store a digital copy for easy updates.

SECTION 7.7: Continence Supplies

Managing continence products effectively prevents unnecessary stress, last-minute shortages and potential health risks. With a structured system in place, caregivers can confidently navigate this aspect of care with ease and compassion.

What This System Covers:

- Understanding different types of continence products and selecting the right ones
- Managing supply levels to avoid shortages
- Preventing infections and maintaining hygiene
- Ensuring dignity and comfort for your loved one
- Training caregivers on proper usage and disposal of supplies

How to Set Up an Effective System:

1. **Assess Your Loved One's Continence Needs**
   Different continence products serve different purposes. Assess whether pads, pull-ups, all-in-ones or catheters are the best fit based on mobility, frequency and comfort. Consulting a healthcare professional may help determine the most suitable products.

2. **Create a Tracking System for Supplies**
   Running out of continence supplies at the wrong moment can lead to stress and discomfort. Implement a simple tracking system – this could be a spreadsheet, a whiteboard checklist or an app – to monitor daily usage and ensure timely reordering.

3. **Implement a Hygiene and Infection Control Plan**
   Proper hygiene prevents infections and skin issues. Ensure caregivers follow a clear protocol for changing products,

cleaning the skin and using barrier creams when necessary. Disposable gloves, wipes and sanitising sprays should be readily available as part of the system.

4. **Design an Accessible and Discreet Storage System**
Continence supplies should be easy to access but stored discreetly. Consider labelled storage bins in a designated cupboard or a bedside organiser for night-time use. Maintaining an organised storage space reduces stress and ensures quick access when needed.

5. **Provide Training and Guidance for Caregivers**
Continence care is a sensitive task and maintaining the dignity of your loved one is paramount. Caregivers should be trained on:

- How to change products safely and comfortably
- Communication techniques to reduce embarrassment
- Proper disposal methods to maintain hygiene and odour control

Action Steps:

- ✓ Educate caregivers on infection control and comfort measures. Refer to *WORKBOOK 7.7: Setting up an effective Continence Supply System Checklist*
- ✓ Set up a structured storage system for easy access and organisation
- ✓ Maintain a weekly supply checklist to track stock levels and prevent shortages. Refer to *WORKBOOK 7.7: Supply Tracking Checklist*
- ✓ Establish a routine for product changes and hygiene to ensure consistency

WORKBOOK 7.7: Setting Up an Effective Continence Supply System

Use this checklist to ensure all aspects of continence care are managed effectively. Tick off each step as you implement or complete it. This system helps prevent infections, maintain dignity and streamline continence care.

☑ Assess Your Loved One's Continence Needs
- ☐ Identify whether pads, pull-ups, all-in-ones or catheters are the most suitable product.
- ☐ Consider mobility, frequency of changes and comfort level when selecting products.
- ☐ Consult a healthcare professional if unsure about the best option.

☑ Create a Supply Tracking System
- ☐ Set up a spreadsheet, checklist or app to track usage and reordering needs.
- ☐ Monitor daily usage rates to predict when stock will run low.
- ☐ Schedule reminders for reordering to avoid last-minute shortages.

☑ Implement a Hygiene and Infection Control Plan
- ☐ Ensure caregivers wash hands thoroughly before and after continence care.
- ☐ Use disposable gloves and change them between tasks.
- ☐ Establish a routine for skin care, including cleansing and barrier creams.
- ☐ Keep disinfecting wipes or sprays nearby to clean surfaces after each change.

☑ Design an Accessible and Discreet Storage System
- ☐ Store continence products in a dry, clean location that is easy to access.

- ☐ Use labelled storage containers or a bedside organiser for quick retrieval.
- ☐ Keep extra supplies out of sight for discretion but within reach for ease of use.

✓ Provide Training for Caregivers

- ☐ Educate caregivers on how to change products safely and comfortably.
- ☐ Teach proper disposal techniques to maintain hygiene.
- ☐ Train caregivers to communicate sensitively to maintain dignity.
- ☐ Reinforce the importance of infection control and skin protection measures.

Supply Tracking Checklist

Consider using a checklist to track continence supplies, monitor stock levels and ensure timely reordering. Regularly updating this tally helps prevent shortages and ensures that continence care runs smoothly.

Date Checked	Product Name	Type (Pads/ Pull-ups/ Catheters)	Quantity in Stock	Daily Usage Rate	Reorder Date

SECTION 7.8: Cleaning and Hygiene

Maintaining a clean and hygienic environment is essential for the health and well-being of both caregivers and their loved ones. A structured system for cleaning and hygiene not only prevents infections but also reduces stress by ensuring tasks are completed consistently and efficiently. By creating an organised approach to cleanliness, caregivers can foster a sense of calm and comfort in their daily routines.

What This System Covers:

- Establishing personal and household cleaning routines
- Preventing infection risks through proper hygiene practices
- Managing cleaning supplies and safe storage
- Creating a structured schedule for maintaining cleanliness
- Educating caregivers on best hygiene practices

How to Set Up an Effective System:

1. Develop a Manageable Cleaning Schedule
A structured yet flexible cleaning schedule ensures a consistently hygienic living environment while keeping tasks manageable. This schedule should include:

- **Daily Tasks:** Light surface wiping, disinfecting high-touch areas, handwashing routines and personal hygiene practices

- **Weekly Tasks:** Refreshing bed linens and towels, vacuuming, mopping floors and deep-cleaning bathrooms

- **Monthly Tasks:** Decluttering spaces, checking expiration dates on cleaning supplies and deep-cleaning appliances

A visible, easy-to-follow checklist can bring reassurance and a sense of accomplishment.

2. Implement a Thoughtful Supply Tracking System

Keeping track of essential cleaning supplies ensures that caregivers never run out at crucial moments. Setting up an effective monitoring system prevents shortages and helps maintain peace of mind. Consider:

- A written checklist
- A well-organised, labelled storage area for quick access to supplies, lockable for safety
- Automated reordering for essential items like disinfectants, gloves and wipes

An organised supply system allows caregivers to focus on providing care rather than worrying about running out of essentials.

3. Provide Training on Infection Control

A structured approach to hygiene protects both the caregiver and the loved one. Training should focus on:

- Effective handwashing techniques with warm water and mild soap
- Disinfection of frequently touched surfaces like door handles, light switches and mobility aids
- Safe and hygienic waste disposal methods for tissues, gloves and continence products
- The proper use of Personal Protective Equipment (PPE) when needed

Ongoing learning and refreshers help caregivers feel confident and prepared in their daily routines.

4. Design a Safe and Organised Storage System for Cleaning Products

Cleaning products should be stored safely to prevent accidents while remaining easily accessible. Consider:

- Lockable cabinets for hazardous chemicals to ensure safety
- Clearly labelled storage bins to make identifying supplies effortless
- Senior-friendly or childproof designs that match household need

By keeping cleaning supplies organised and accessible, caregivers can maintain a structured and safe home environment.

Action Steps:

- ✓ Create a weekly and monthly cleaning checklist using *WORKBOOK 7.8: Cleaning Routine Checklist*
- ✓ Maintain an easy-to-follow inventory list of cleaning and hygiene supplies for purchasing needs using *WORKBOOK 7.8: Cleaning Product Inventory Checklist*
- ✓ Provide structured training on hygiene best practices and infection control
- ✓ Take steps to prevent infection risks and cross-contamination using *WORKBOOK 7.8: Cleaning Routine Checklist*

WORKBOOK 7.8: Cleaning Routine Checklist

☑ **Daily Cleaning Tasks:**
- ☐ Wipe down and disinfect high-touch surfaces (e.g., door handles, light switches, remotes, handrails)
- ☐ Clean kitchen surfaces and sinks
- ☐ Wash used dishes or load dishwasher
- ☐ Take out rubbish and replace bin liners
- ☐ Sweep or vacuum high-traffic areas
- ☐ Ensure bathroom surfaces remain dry and clean
- ☐ Wash laundry, hang out to dry and fold back into the cupboard
- ☐ Encourage and maintain personal hygiene routines

☑ **Weekly Cleaning Tasks:**
- ☐ Mop floors and vacuum carpets thoroughly
- ☐ Change and wash bed linens and towels
- ☐ Disinfect and deep-clean bathroom surfaces
- ☐ Wipe down kitchen appliances and cupboards
- ☐ Dust furniture, shelves and baseboards
- ☐ Clean inside the fridge and discard expired food
- ☐ Launder frequently used fabrics such as cushion covers and hand towels

☑ **Monthly Cleaning Tasks:**
- ☐ Deep-clean under furniture and appliances
- ☐ Declutter storage areas and dispose of unnecessary items
- ☐ Wash windows and wipe down window sills
- ☐ Rotate and check expiration dates on cleaning products
- ☐ Organise and sanitise cleaning supply storage areas
- ☐ Wash and disinfect bins and waste disposal units

☑ **Preventing Infection and Cross-Contamination:**
- ☐ Wash hands regularly for at least 20 seconds with soap and warm water.

- ☐ Use separate cleaning cloths and sponges for different areas (e.g., kitchen vs. bathroom).
- ☐ Avoid cross-contamination by disinfecting high-touch surfaces multiple times a day.
- ☐ Properly dispose of soiled tissues, gloves and hygiene products.
- ☐ Launder bed linens and towels at high temperatures to kill germs.
- ☐ Keep cleaning supplies in a designated storage area to avoid contamination.
- ☐ Use PPE when handling waste or cleaning bodily fluids to reduce infection risk.
- ☐ Educate caregivers on best practices for maintaining cleanliness and hygiene.

WORKBOOK 7.8: Cleaning Product Inventory Checklist

Tick the item to be purchased:

Category	Item	☑
Disinfectants and Surface Cleaners	Multi-purpose disinfectant spray	[ ]
	Antibacterial wipes	[ ]
	Bleach or hospital-grade disinfectant	[ ]
	Glass cleaner	[ ]
Bathroom and Toilet Supplies	Toilet bowl cleaner	[ ]
	Mould and mildew remover	[ ]
	Shower and tile cleaner	[ ]
	Bathroom air freshener	[ ]
	Disposable toilet brushes	[ ]
	Sink and drain cleaner	[ ]
Floor and Carpet Cleaners	Mop and bucket	[ ]
	Floor disinfectant or cleaner	[ ]
	Vacuum cleaner bags/ filters	[ ]
	Carpet stain remover	[ ]
	Wood floor polish	[ ]
	Steam mop	[ ]

Category	Item	✔
Laundry and Fabric Care	Laundry detergent	[ ]
	Fabric softener	[ ]
	Stain remover	[ ]
	Disposable gloves for handling soiled laundry	[ ]
	Mesh laundry bags	[ ]
	Ironing spray	[ ]
Personal Protective Equipment	Disposable gloves	[ ]
	Face masks	[ ]
	Hand sanitiser	[ ]
	Protective aprons	[ ]
	Safety goggles	[ ]
Waste Management	Rubbish bags	[ ]
	Recycling bin liners	[ ]
	Biohazard waste bags	[ ]
	Compostable bags	[ ]
	Odour-neutralising bin deodoriser	[ ]

Notes: ____

SECTION 7.9: Staffing and Support Networks

Caregiving is not a solo journey. Whether you're relying on professional support staff, family members or a combination of both, having a structured staffing and support network ensures continuity, reduces burnout and improves the quality of care. A strong system helps you recruit the right people, train them effectively and maintain smooth operations even when primary caregivers are unavailable.

A well-organised support network means everyone involved understands their role, follows clear guidelines and works as a team to provide the best care possible. By setting up structured recruitment, training and communication processes, you create a reliable and sustainable caregiving system.

Refer to the workbook at the end of this chapter: *WORKBOOK 7.9: Staffing and Support Networks Checklist*

What This System Covers:

- Recruiting, training and managing support staff effectively
- Developing a structured onboarding and training process
- Establishing clear communication and boundaries with caregivers
- Creating a scheduling system for caregiver shifts
- Ensuring continuity of care when primary caregivers are unavailable

How to Set Up an Effective System:

1. Develop a Hiring and Screening Process to Find Qualified, Compassionate Staff

Recruiting the right caregivers is about more than just qualifications – it's about trust, reliability and shared values. Your support staff will play a critical role in your loved one's daily care, so taking the time to properly screen, train and select the right individuals is essential for long-term stability and quality care. To make this process manageable, we will break it into five key steps:

1. **Define the Role and Expectations** – Understand what kind of care is needed.

2. **Develop a Recruitment Strategy** – Identify the best sources for finding caregivers.

3. **Screen Candidates Thoroughly** – Use structured interviews, reference checks and background screening.

4. **Conduct a Trial Shift** – Observe the candidate's real-life caregiving skills.

5. **Offer Employment and Set Clear Expectations** – Formalise the hiring process with agreements and onboarding.

By following these steps, you can ensure that only the most capable and compassionate caregivers become part of your support team.

Step 1: Define the Role and Expectations

The first step in building a strong support network is planning this stage with your loved one. Wherever possible, they should have input, choices and a say in who provides their care. This ensures that the support is tailored to their personality, needs and comfort level, rather than simply filling a vacancy.

It's also important to consider factors like gender and age appropriateness when selecting a support worker. A well-matched caregiver enhances the quality of care, builds trust and improves overall well-being. For example, if you are hiring support for a teenage boy who enjoys sports and video games, he may feel more comfortable and engaged with a like-minded male support worker who shares his interests, rather than someone he struggles to relate to.

By involving your loved one in the decision-making process, you ensure that the support provided is not only practical but also emotionally and socially meaningful. Before beginning the hiring process, take time to identify exactly what type of support is needed. Consider:

- **Work hours and flexibility** – Will support be required daily, overnight or just a few times a week? Is flexibility needed for medical appointments or social outings?
- **Formal qualifications and training** – Depending on the level of care required, you may prefer a support worker who has relevant certifications such as Certificate III or IV in Disability, Aged Care or Individual Support, First Aid and CPR, Manual Handling or Medication Assistance Training.
- **Specialised training** – Does the caregiver need experience with specific conditions like dementia, autism, diabetes or complex physical disabilities?
- **Personality match** – Does your loved one prefer a chatty and social caregiver or someone who is more quiet and reserved?
- **Soft skills** – Traits like patience, empathy, reliability and clear communication are just as important as experience.

Once these expectations are clearly defined, it becomes much easier to screen candidates and find the right fit for your loved one's care. This planning step lays the foundation for a smooth and effective hiring process, ensuring that your support network is reliable, compassionate and aligned with your loved one's needs and preferences.

The next step is to find the right candidates who meet your loved one's needs. A well-thought-out recruitment strategy helps attract skilled, reliable and compassionate caregivers while ensuring you have a structured approach to hiring.

Unlike traditional job searches, hiring a caregiver requires more than just checking qualifications – it's about finding someone who is the right fit for your loved one's personality, routine and care needs. A good recruitment strategy ensures that the hiring process is efficient, thorough and results in a support network you can trust.

Step 2: Where to Find Caregivers
Depending on your situation, there are several ways to recruit caregivers:

- **Word of mouth and personal recommendation**s – Trusted referrals from friends, family or other caregivers can be a great way to find reliable support.
- **Professional caregiver agencies** – These agencies often have pre-screened, qualified staff who are experienced in working with individuals who require extra support.
- **Online caregiver networks and job boards** – Platforms like *Mable, Hireup, Careseekers* or *NDIS* provider directories can help connect you with independent support workers. Also Facebook and LinkedIn platforms allow joining groups and advertise.
- **Community and disability support organisations** – Local carer groups, disability networks or respite care services often have recommendations for available caregivers.
- **Government-funded home care and NDIS providers** – If your loved one receives government support, working with registered providers can ensure access to qualified caregivers who meet safety and quality standards.

Note for Sole Traders: You may choose to engage a private support worker who operates independently. These individuals often offer more flexible arrangements and can provide a more personalised approach, though it's important to carry out your own screening and agreements to ensure suitability and safety. A combination of these methods may be the most effective way to find the right fit for your loved one's care.

Step 3: Creating a Job Advertisement
If you are directly hiring a caregiver, you may need to create a job listing to attract applicants. A well-written job advertisement should be:

- Clear and specific – Outline the exact tasks, expectations and any specialised skills required.
- Engaging – Caregiving is a person-centred role, so describe the type of person who would be the best fit for the position.
- Honest about working conditions – Be upfront about hours, responsibilities, flexibility and any physical demands.
- Professional but warm – A caregiver is not just an employee but a support partner, so ensure the listing reflects your family's values and the level of trust required in the role.

Here's an example of a job ad:

Seeking a Compassionate Support Worker for In-Home Care
We are looking for a caring, reliable support worker to assist a 45-year-old woman with daily living tasks, social outings and personal care. The ideal candidate will be patient, friendly and have experience working with individuals with mobility challenges. Duties include personal care, meal preparation, companionship and transport assistance. Shifts available: Monday-Friday, 8am-3pm. Requirements: Certificate IV in Disability, First Aid, CPR and Police check and NDIS Worker Screening certificate. Mobility and hoisting training is a must!

If you are using an agency, they will typically handle this step for you by matching available caregivers with your specific needs.

Here's another example for a job ad:

<u>*Seeking a Private Sole Trader Support Worker for In-Home Care*</u>
Location: *[Insert Suburb/City]*
Hours: *Specify if the hours are flexible, casual or part-time, depending on your needs*
Rate: *Negotiable based on experience and qualifications (optional)*

We are looking for an experienced independent support worker (sole trader) to provide personalised care and assistance for [loved one's name or description, e.g., an elderly parent, individual with a disability, recovering patient]. The ideal candidate will be compassionate, reliable and able to work independently while providing high-quality care.

Key Responsibilities:
- *Assisting with daily living tasks, including meal preparation and personal care.*
- *Providing companionship and emotional support.*
- *Transporting to appointments, shopping and community activities.*
- *Administering medications as per care plan (if required).*
- *Supporting exercise programs and therapy routines.*
- *Maintaining clear and professional communication with family members and healthcare professionals.*

Essential Requirements:
- *Must have an ABN, own Public Liability and Professional Indemnity Insurance.*
- *Current First Aid and CPR Certificate.*
- *Police check and NDIS Worker Screening (or willingness to obtain).*
- *Relevant qualifications in Aged Care, Disability or Individual Support (preferred but not essential).*

- *Administration of medication.*
- *Experience working in home care, disability support or aged care.*
- *Reliable transport and a valid driver's licence.*
- *Strong communication and interpersonal skills.*

Why Join Us?
- *Work directly with a family in a private home setting.*
- *Flexible hours with a supportive environment.*
- *Opportunity to build a long-term, one-on-one caregiving relationship.*

How to Apply:
If you are an independent support worker looking to provide personalised, high-quality care, we would love to hear from you. Please email your resume, cover letter and proof of sole trader status (ABN) to [Insert Contact Email] or call [Insert Phone Number] for more details.

Applications will be reviewed as they are received. Thank you for your interest!

This ad ensures clarity on sole trader requirements, promotes flexibility and highlights the personal, one-on-one caregiving relationship – a key benefit for private workers seeking independent clients.

Step 4: Screen Candidates Thoroughly

A structured interview and screening process ensures you hire caregivers who align with your values and needs. An interview should focus on:

- Experience in caregiving and working with similar conditions.
- Problem-solving skills: Ask how they would handle specific situations, such as a loved one refusing medication.

- Communication and interpersonal skills: Can they explain things clearly and listen attentively?

Essential Pre-Employment Checks:

☐ Reference checks: Speak with previous employers or clients to verify experience and reliability.

☐ Background checks: Ensure police check, working with children check clearances and *NDIS* Worker Screening checks are completed.

☐ First Aid and CPR Certification: Verify that candidates are prepared for medical emergencies.

☐ Manual handling and medication training: If required, confirm they have training in safe mobility assistance and administering medications.

This step ensures that only well-qualified, trustworthy caregivers are considered for employment.

Conducting a Trial Shift

Once you have a strong candidate, consider offering a trial shift before making a final decision.

- Observe how they interact with your loved one – are they patient, kind and respectful?
- Assess whether they follow care instructions and adapt to routines.
- Notice if they engage positively or seem disengaged and distracted.

A trial shift allows you to see them in action and ensure they are a good fit both practically and personally.

Step 5: Offer Employment and Set Clear Expectations
After selecting the ideal caregiver, it's crucial to formalise the employment arrangement and establish clear guidelines to ensure a harmonious working relationship. This process involves:

Drafting a Comprehensive Employment Agreement
A written contract serves as a foundational document that outlines the terms and conditions of employment, helping to prevent misunderstandings. An agreement is only essential if the support staff is a sole trader and privately hired. Key components include:

- **Duties and Responsibilities:** Clearly define the caregiver's tasks, such as personal care, meal preparation, medication management and any other specific duties.

- **Work Hours and Schedule:** Specify working days, hours and any expectations regarding flexibility or overtime.

- **Compensation:** Detail the agreed-upon wage, payment frequency and any benefits or reimbursements.

- **Employment Status:** Indicate whether the caregiver is an employee or an independent contractor, as this affects your tax obligations and legal responsibilities.

- **Termination Conditions:** Outline the circumstances under which either party can terminate the agreement, including required notice periods.

For reference, sample caregiver contracts are available, such as *Poppins Payroll*.

Implementing a Structured Training and Onboarding Process
A well-organised onboarding process helps the caregiver acclimate

to their new role and understand your expectations. Consider the following steps:

- **Orientation:** Introduce the support worker to your home environment, household members and any specific equipment or tools they will use, including introducing them to the work instructions and protocols to follow.

- **Shadowing Period:** Allow the new support worker to observe and assist existing caregivers or family members to learn established routines and preferences. Give them time to adjust, learn and feel comfortable before working with our loved one on their own.

- **Ongoing Support:** Provide opportunities for regular feedback and open communication to address any questions or concerns.

- Implementing a structured onboarding process not only enhances caregiver performance but also improves retention rates. By formalising the employment relationship and setting clear expectations from the outset, you lay the groundwork for a positive and productive partnership, ensuring your loved one receives consistent and compassionate care.

Establishing Clear Communication and Boundaries

Good communication prevents misunderstandings and ensures everyone is on the same page.

- **Set clear expectations early** – Outline written instructions, protocols and daily routines, medical needs and house rules in a way that is easy to follow. Equip the support worker with comprehensive care plans that detail daily routines, medical requirements, dietary preferences and emergency protocols. This ensures consistency and quality of care.

- **Encourage open dialogue** – Regular check-ins help address concerns before they become problems. Create a space where the support worker feels comfortable raising issues or asking for guidance.

- **Respect personal and professional boundaries** – Support workers need to feel valued but not overwhelmed. Ensure work-life balance is maintained to prevent burnout. Likewise expect respect in return.

Example: If your loved one prefers quiet time in the afternoon, let caregivers know so they can structure activities around this rather than pushing for engagement when rest is needed.

Creating a Scheduling System for Caregiver Shifts
Consistency is crucial in caregiving and well-organised schedules help prevent gaps in care.

- **Create a weekly roster** that factors in regular support workers, backup staff and time off to avoid burnout.

- **Use scheduling tools** like simple printed timetables, spreadsheets, whiteboards or care apps can help caregivers and family members coordinate shifts. Certainly, some caregiver scheduling applications I've come across include *ShiftCare, RosterElf, Deputy, Connecteam* and *Skedulo.*

- **Factor in flexibility** for unforeseen circumstances may require last-minute adjustments, so have a system where carers can swap shifts or provide cover when needed.

Example: If your loved one needs overnight supervision but their usual carer is unavailable, having a standby list of pre-approved, trained caregivers ensures they are never left without support.

Ensuring continuity of care when primary support workers are unavailable

Planning for flexibility in caregiver scheduling is essential, especially during long weekends, public holidays and annual celebrations like Christmas, as these events can disrupt regular shift patterns. To manage this effectively:

- **Plan Ahead:** Anticipate upcoming holidays and special occasions by creating schedules well in advance. This proactive approach allows you to arrange your personal plans accordingly and ensures that all shifts are adequately covered. Also by asking the support workers to give as much notice as possible for their time off/ annual holidays.

- **Accommodate Caregiver Preferences:** Recognise that support workers may have personal commitments during these periods. By considering their availability and preferences, you can foster goodwill and reduce the likelihood of last-minute absences.

- **Implement a Shift-Swapping System:** Establish a clear protocol that enables staff to exchange shifts among themselves, provided all parties agree and the quality of care remains consistent. This system offers flexibility and empowers caregivers to manage their schedules collaboratively.

- **Maintain a Pool of Backup Caregivers:** Having a list of trained, on-call staff ready to step in during unforeseen circumstances ensures that care is uninterrupted, even when primary caregivers are unavailable.

By integrating these strategies, you can create a resilient scheduling system that adapts to both planned events and unexpected changes, ensuring continuous and reliable care for your loved one and to yourself.

Action Steps:

✓ Develop a hiring and screening process
✓ Establish clear communication and boundaries
✓ Develop a structured onboarding and training process
✓ Create a scheduling system for caregiver shifts
✓ Ensure continuity of care when primary caregivers are unavailable

Refer to *WORKBOOK 7.9: Staffing and Support Networks Checklist for all these action steps*

WORKBOOK 7.9: Staffing and Support Networks Checklist

Use this checklist to build a structured caregiver support system that ensures smooth recruitment, training, scheduling and communication. Tick off each task as you complete it.

✔	Action Steps	Tasks to Complete	✔
☐	**Develop a Hiring and Screening Process**	Define required skills, qualifications and personal traits.	☐
		Write a clear job description.	☐
		Advertise through caregiver agencies, job boards or word of mouth.	☐
		Conduct interviews with a mix of situational and experience-based questions.	☐
		Perform background checks, verify references and confirm necessary certifications.	☐
		Shortlist candidates and arrange a trial shift before final selection.	☐
☐	**Establish Clear Communication and Boundaries**	Set clear expectations for tasks, working hours and responsibilities.	☐
		Encourage open and ongoing communication between caregivers and family members.	☐
		Provide a structured method for shift handovers (e.g., written logs or verbal updates).	☐
		Maintain professional boundaries to ensure a respectful working environment.	☐
		Offer regular feedback and support to caregivers.	☐
☐	**Develop a Structured Onboarding and Training Process**	Provide an orientation session introducing the home environment, household members and care routines.	☐

✔	Action Steps	Tasks to Complete	✔
		Supply written care plans outlining daily tasks, medical needs and emergency protocols.	☐
		Ensure caregivers receive training in manual handling, medication administration and first aid.	☐
		Implement a shadowing period where new caregivers observe experienced staff before working independently.	☐
		Conduct regular refresher training to keep caregivers updated on best practices.	☐
☐	**Create a Scheduling System for Caregiver Shifts**	Develop a structured weekly or monthly roster ensuring adequate coverage.	☐
		Use scheduling tools or software to coordinate shifts.	☐
		Plan for holiday periods and celebrations, allowing caregivers time off while ensuring adequate cover.	☐
		Have a shift-swapping system in place to manage last-minute adjustments.	☐
☐	**Ensure Continuity of Care When Primary Caregivers Are Unavailable**	Cross-train multiple caregivers so they are familiar with essential routines.	☐
		Maintain a list of backup caregivers who can step in when needed.	☐
		Keep all care plans and work instructions updated and easily accessible.	☐
		Ensure all caregivers know emergency contacts and procedures for medical incidents.	☐

SECTION 7.10: Emergency Preparedness and Fire Safety

Emergencies don't send invitations – they arrive unannounced, demanding quick action. As a caregiver, being prepared for the unexpected means ensuring the safety of both you and your loved one. Whether it's a sudden fire, a power outage or a medical crisis, having a solid plan in place can mean the difference between chaos and calm. This chapter will guide you in creating a structured system to handle emergencies efficiently and keep your caregiving environment safe.

What This System Covers:

- Developing an emergency response plan tailored to your loved one's needs, including house fires.
- Preparing for fire, medical emergencies and power outages.
- Ensuring a safe environment through fire safety and prevention measures.
- Keeping an up-to-date emergency contact list and communication strategy, along with having personal documents ready to grab in an emergency.
- Assembling and maintaining an emergency kit with essential supplies.

How to Set Up an Effective System:

1. **Assess the Risks:** Take a moment to reflect on the specific risks your loved one might face. Does your loved one rely on medical equipment that needs electricity? Are there mobility challenges that could make an evacuation difficult? Consider daily routines – what areas might be at higher risk for fires or emergencies? Talking through these possibilities with your loved one and other caregivers can help you feel more prepared and less overwhelmed.

2. **Plan Your Response:** Creating a plan isn't about focusing on fear – it's about building confidence. Work together with your loved one to create a simple, easy-to-follow emergency response plan.

   - Walk through the home and identify the safest exits for different types of emergencies.
   - Consider accessibility and energy levels– how will your loved one move quickly and safely?
   - Assign roles within your caregiving network – who, when and how calls for help? Who, when and how assists in evacuation?
   - Create a written copy of emergency contacts and procedures and keep them in multiple locations.
   - If possible, practice the plan together so that it feels familiar and manageable.

3. **Build Your Emergency Kit:** A well-prepared emergency kit is crucial in ensuring that you and your loved one can respond effectively in a crisis and can evacuate with having an emergency kit that is easy to grab on the go. Start with the basics – water, non- perishable foods, medications, a torch, spare chargers and important documents. These are fundamental to survival in situations where power or resources may be cut off. However, beyond the basics, consider the specific needs of your loved one.

   If they rely on medications, ensure you have at least a week's supply readily available, along with a copy of their prescriptions and medical documents such as a medical folder. For those with mobility challenges, think beyond just medication – wheelchair users may need an extra cushion for comfort, spare batteries if using an electric wheelchair or a manual alternative in case power is unavailable. If hoists are used, having a manual hoist on hand can be invaluable should electric equipment fail.

Comfort items should not be overlooked. In an emergency, having familiar objects, such as a favourite blanket or a stress-relief toy, can help ease anxiety. Also, consider communication – have a written emergency contacts list, ensuring that important numbers are easily accessible if mobile devices fail. If your loved one uses electronic medical devices, a backup power source or battery-operated alternatives should be part of your kit.

Keeping a small version of your emergency kit in the car adds another layer of preparedness, ensuring you're never caught off guard when away from home.

4. **Fire Safety Essentials:** Fire safety is more than just having smoke alarms – it's about creating a safe environment every day.

   - Keep walkways clear to ensure an easy exit in case of an emergency.
   - If your loved one uses oxygen, store it safely away from open flames.
   - Establish a 'safe zone' in the kitchen where hot surfaces and flames are avoided.
   - Never leave cooking unattended, and always switch off power points, lights, and appliances when they're not in use. Regularly check that fire extinguishers, smoke alarms and escape routes are in good condition. Prepare a simple emergency plan that others can easily follow – having clear steps on hand can provide guidance during stressful or chaotic situations.
   - Draw a floor plan of your home and mark the locations of fire alarms, fire blankets, fire extinguishers,

emergency kit, and all available exits for quick reference.

- Teach your loved one and any other caregivers how to use a fire extinguisher – it's a skill that can save lives.

5. **Practice Makes Prepared:** Emergencies can feel chaotic but practice can reduce panic and make responses feel second nature. It's important to ensure that all caregivers, including family members, friends and support workers, are familiar with emergency procedures and protocols. New supports should be inducted into the emergency plan as soon as they begin assisting in caregiving.

Note: For detailed guidance on fire prevention, preparedness, and home safety planning, refer to reputable sources such as the Country Fire Authority (CFA) website in your state. (Australia only)

This includes reviewing the emergency response plan, walking through escape routes and demonstrating how to use fire safety equipment. Clear communication and regular refreshers ensure that everyone is on the same page and ready to act swiftly when needed.

If your loved one has mobility restrictions, it's essential to prepare for how to safely assist them during an emergency. Caregivers should be trained on how to use different equipment, such as wheelchairs, hoists and transfer aids, ensuring that these are easily accessible and in good working order. If your home relies on ceiling hoists or other powered mobility devices, always have a manual backup option available in case of a power outage. Keeping a torch or emergency lighting nearby can be useful if evacuations need to take place in low visibility. Additionally, have a backup plan for medical equipment that requires electricity, such as oxygen machines or feeding pumps, ensuring that battery-operated alternatives or a portable power source are readily available.

- Set reminders to review and update your plan every six months.
- If your loved one struggles with anxiety around emergencies, ease into preparedness conversations slowly.
- Role-play small scenarios to help everyone feel more confident.
- Don't forget to reward efforts – turn drills into small celebrations to create a sense of accomplishment rather than fear.

Action Steps:

- ✓ Install and check fire safety equipment, such as smoke alarms and extinguishers
- ✓ Create a written emergency plan and share it with all caregivers. Refer to *WORKBOOK 7.10: Quick Emergency Guide*
- ✓ Maintain an emergency supply kit tailored to medical needs
- ✓ Conduct fire safety and emergency drills every six months
- ✓ Stay informed about local emergency services and available support

WORKBOOK 7.10: Quick Emergency Guide

What to Do, What to Grab and Getting Your Loved One Out

Step 1: Stay Calm and Assess the Situation
- Take a deep breath and quickly determine the nature of the emergency.
- Follow Protocols and Written Instructions for guidance
- If it's a power outage, ensure your loved one is safe and secure before taking action. Use torch and other prepared items such as batteries for medical equipment while the power is out. Check local services on your mobile to find out the nature and duration of the power outage.
- If there is a fire, feel doors for heat before opening and stay low if there's smoke. Investigate the nature and severity of fire. (only if safe to do so)

Fire Situation
Step 2: Alert and Evacuate
- Sound an alarm if necessary and alert anyone in the home.
- Try to put out any small fires (only of safe to do so).
- Help your loved one move to the nearest identified exit (refer to your home diagram).
- If evacuation is not possible, get to a safe area and call emergency services immediately. In Australia, it is '000' for Fire, Ambulance and Police.

Step 3: Grab Essential Items (Only If Safe to Do So)
- Your grab-and-go emergency bag/ kit (medications, medical documents, water, phone charger).
- Any mobility aids or medical equipment your loved one needs.
- Emergency contacts list and any pre-prepared personal documents.

Step 4: Get to the Assembly Point

- Move to your designated safe meeting place (e.g., neighbour's driveway, in a park across the road).
- Account for everyone and contact emergency services if you haven't already.
- Stay together and follow emergency personnel instructions.

Step 5: Check In and Provide Comfort

- Ensure your loved one is comfortable and reassure them that help is on the way.
- If needed, use any medical supplies from your emergency kit until help arrives.
- Contact family members or caregivers to update them on the situation.
- Do not go back in the house, until emergency personnel states it is safe to do so.

SECTION 7.11: Transport Obligations

Getting your loved one from place to place safely and comfortably is more than just arranging a ride – it's about ensuring their safety, independence, dignity and well-being. Whether it's a doctor's visit, a social outing or simply a change of scenery, having a reliable transport system in place can take a huge weight off your shoulders.

This chapter helps you put together a plan that makes transport easier and stress-free, from finding the right vehicle to managing schedules and setting boundaries for safety. It also touches on the importance of training caregivers in safe transfers and making sure drivers and vehicles meet the right standards.

While transport can sometimes feel like a logistical puzzle, with the right system, it becomes just another smooth part of the caregiving journey – helping your loved one stay connected to the world while giving you peace of mind.

What This System Covers:

- Planning and arranging safe and accessible transport for medical appointments and daily activities.
- Ensuring compliance with mobility needs, including wheelchair-accessible vehicles.
- Managing transport logistics, schedules and backup plans.
- Training caregivers and loved ones on safe vehicle entry and exit techniques.
- Identifying available transport services and funding options.
- Ensuring driver's vehicle compliance.
- Setting clear transport boundaries to avoid unnecessary detours or unapproved outings.

How to Set Up an Effective System:

1. **Plan Safe and Accessible Transport**
   Ensuring that transportation arrangements are reliable and suitable for your loved one's mobility needs is essential. This includes scheduling trips for medical appointments, daily activities and social outings while maintaining an organised and conflict-free transport plan. A shared calendar accessible to caregivers helps to coordinate trips effectively and prevent missed appointments.

2. **Meet Mobility Needs**
   Vehicles used for transport must be equipped to accommodate any required mobility aids, such as wheelchairs or walking frames. Caregivers and drivers should be trained in handling and securing these aids properly to ensure comfort and safety during travel. Regular checks should be conducted to confirm the suitability and maintenance of accessibility features in the vehicle.

3. **Manage Transport Logistics**
   A well-organised transport system helps prevent last-minute stress. This includes coordinating trip schedules, maintaining flexibility for sudden changes and having a backup plan in place to ensure smooth and hassle-free travel arrangements. Identifying alternative transport options such as community transport services or rideshare programs designed for people with disabilities is useful in case of disruptions.

4. **Train on Safe Transfers**
   Caregivers and loved ones should be trained in safe vehicle entry and exit techniques to minimise the risk of injury. Proper seatbelt use, adjusting restraints and following accessibility protocols make transport safer for everyone

involved. Training sessions should include demonstrations on correct lifting techniques and securing mobility devices. Every vehicle is different, so it's important to include practice sessions with your support worker and loved one on the safest and most comfortable way to enter and exit the vehicle as part of your training and induction process.

5. **Explore Transport Services**

Researching and registering for government-funded and private transport assistance programs can help ease financial burdens. Accessible community transport options should also be considered to expand mobility choices. Consider applying for a Taxi Subsidy Scheme as a backup option to reduce the stress of finding alternative transport in unexpected situations or emergencies. (See Chapter 5 for details). Keeping a list of reliable services, their costs and availability ensures alternative arrangements can be made when needed. These can be summarised in a QR code for other supports to scan by their mobile and refer to for assistance.

6. **Ensure Driver and Vehicle Compliance**

Before allowing anyone to transport your loved one, request proof of a valid driver's licence, vehicle registration and full insurance coverage. Keeping this information on file allows for periodic reviews to ensure compliance and continued safety. It is your right to verify that any vehicle being used is roadworthy and appropriately insured to cover potential incidents.

7. **Set Clear Transport Boundaries**

Your loved one's transport should always be planned and approved by you. Avoiding unnecessary detours, visits to unfamiliar locations or social outings with support workers' friends ensures safety and comfort at all times. If a trip outside of pre-approved locations is required, prior consent must be obtained from you to ensure transparency and accountability.

Action Steps:

- ✓ Use *WORKBOOK 7.11: Transport Obligations Checklist* to complete the following steps:
- ✓ Develop a transport schedule that aligns with medical and social needs
- ✓ Research and document accessible transport options in the local area
- ✓ Train caregivers on safe transfer techniques for individuals with mobility challenges
- ✓ Verify the credentials of any individual transporting your loved one
- ✓ Establish written guidelines on transport safety
- ✓ Communicate safety expectations with caregivers, ensuring no unexpected detours or unauthorised social visits

WORKBOOK 7.11: Transport Obligations Checklist

☑ Planning and Scheduling
- ☐ Create a transport schedule for medical appointments and social activities
- ☐ Share the schedule with caregivers using a calendar or app
- ☐ Plan backup transport options for last-minute changes

☑ Meeting Mobility Needs
- ☐ Confirm the vehicle is accessible for mobility aids (e.g., wheelchair, walking frame)
- ☐ Train caregivers on securing and handling mobility aids during transport
- ☐ Conduct regular checks on accessibility features and safety equipment in the vehicle

☑ Managing Transport Logistics
- ☐ Identify and document available transport services (e.g., community transport, rideshare options)
- ☐ Establish a backup plan in case of schedule disruptions
- ☐ Ensure caregivers and loved ones are aware of the transport plan

☑ Safe Transfers and Training
- ☐ Train caregivers on safe vehicle entry and exit techniques
- ☐ Review seatbelt safety and proper positioning of mobility aids
- ☐ Provide demonstrations on safe lifting techniques for assistance

☑ Exploring Transport Services
- ☐ Research government-funded and private transport programs
- ☐ Keep a list of accessible transport options, costs and contact details
- ☐ Register for any available financial assistance for transport

☑ Driver and Vehicle Compliance
- ☐ Verify the driver has a valid licence and full insurance coverage
- ☐ Ensure the vehicle is registered, roadworthy and properly maintained
- ☐ Keep a record of compliance checks for each transport provider

☑ Setting Transport Boundaries
- ☐ Define and communicate transport rules (e.g., no unapproved stops or detours)
- ☐ Establish clear guidelines for approving transport requests
- ☐ Ensure caregivers understand and follow transport safety expectations

SECTION 7.12: Preparing for Your Holiday as Your Respite

Taking a holiday when you're a caregiver can feel like an impossible task. The worry, the planning and the guilt often make it easier to just push the idea aside. But the truth is, *you need this time away.* Stepping back, even briefl y, isn't just about rest – it's about giving yourself the chance to breathe, reset and return feeling stronger.

A well-prepared break allows you to truly relax, knowing your loved one is safe and well cared for in your absence. With the right steps in place, you can set up a system that supports both you and them – so when you take that first deep breath on holiday, it won't be weighed down by worry.

What This System Covers:

- Planning a holiday while ensuring continuity of care for your loved one
- Identifying temporary caregiving support and respite options
- Preparing support and staffing while away
- Preparing an emergency contact plan for while you are away
- Ensuring self-care and relaxation during your time off

How to Set Up an Effective System:

- **Plan early and confirm your dates.** Start planning as soon as you can – good respite options fill up quickly. Lock in your travel dates and put them on paper. The sooner you commit, the sooner you can start putting support in place.

- **Find and organise temporary caregiving support.** Look at different options: respite care facilities, in-home support workers or a trusted family member. If you're hiring professional help, meet with them beforehand, go through the daily routine and ensure they're comfortable with your loved one's needs. If a friend or family member is stepping in, offer a trial run so they feel confident before you leave.

- **Prepare a detailed care plan and daily guide.** Write down everything – routines, meal preferences, medications, key contacts. The more information your temporary caregiver has, the smoother things will run. Think of it like leaving instructions for a babysitter but with added details on healthcare and emotional needs.

- **Set up an emergency plan.** Identify a primary point of contact who can handle any urgent situations. Leave copies of essential documents – healthcare information, medication lists and emergency numbers – with them. Let your loved one's doctor know about your absence so they can assist if needed.

- **Give yourself permission to switch off.** It's natural to worry but constant check-ins defeat the purpose of your break. Set clear expectations with your temporary caregiver – maybe a daily text update is enough, rather than constant calls. Trust the plan you've put in place and allow yourself to enjoy this well-deserved rest.

Taking time for yourself doesn't mean neglecting your loved one – it means ensuring you can keep showing up for them long-term. When you prepare well, you create the space to recharge, reset and return with a full heart and fresh energy.

Action Steps:

- ✓ Confirm your holiday dates
- ✓ Arrange temporary caregiving support
- ✓ Follow checklist to prepare for the holiday using *WORK-BOOK 7.12: Caregiver's Holiday Preparation Checklist*

WORKBOOK 7.12: Caregiver's Holiday Preparation Checklist

Taking a break as a caregiver requires careful planning to ensure everything runs smoothly in your absence. Use this checklist to prepare your loved one's care, your home and yourself for a stress-free holiday. Tick off each item as you complete it to stay organised.

✓	Task
☐	Confirm travel dates and book necessary arrangements
☐	Arrange temporary caregiving support (respite care, in-home support or family/friends)
☐	Create a detailed daily care plan for your loved one, including routines and medical needs
☐	Prepare an emergency plan and assign a key contact person
☐	Provide temporary caregiver with medical and emergency contacts
☐	Organise a check-in system to stay informed without constant contact
☐	Prepare the house (stock up on essentials organise medications, leave instructions)
☐	Arrange care for pets (pet sitter, boarding or trusted friend)
☐	Pack travel essentials (passport, tickets, medications, comfort items)
☐	Set up automatic bill payments and notify key services of your absence
☐	Leave emergency numbers with a neighbour or close friend

SECTION 7.13: Creating a Safe and Accessible Environment

Your loved one's home should be their sanctuary – a place where they feel safe, comfortable and able to move freely. As a caregiver, ensuring a secure and accessible environment also means reducing risks, preventing injuries and making daily caregiving more manageable.

A well-designed home can enhance both your loved one's independence and your ability to provide effective care, easing the physical and emotional demands of caregiving. It is also important to ensure that the home is safe and accessible for support workers, family members and others who come in to assist. A well-prepared space not only benefits your loved one but also makes it easier for others to provide care and support efficiently and safely.

What This System Covers:

- Ensuring security and accessibility within the home
- Leveraging equipment and assistive devices for safety and ease
- Maintaining a clutter-free and well-organised space
- Responding to injuries and emergency situations at home

By addressing these key areas, you can create a living environment that promotes safety, independence and peace of mind for both you and your loved one.

How to Set Up an Effective System:

1. **Ensuring Security and Accessibility**
   Making a home safer starts with identifying and removing potential hazards. Many accidents occur due to small but preventable risks, such as loose rugs, poor lighting or narrow

doorways. Simple modifications can make a significant difference, such as:

- **Clear pathways and clutter-free spaces:** Ensure hallways, entrances and frequently used areas are free of obstacles. This is particularly important for individuals using mobility aids such as walkers or wheelchairs.
- **Adequate lighting:** Well-lit spaces reduce the risk of falls. Consider installing motion-activated lighting in hallways, bathrooms and staircases for convenience.
- **Grab rails and supports:** Install grab rails in key areas, such as bathrooms, near beds and along staircases. These provide essential stability and support, reducing the strain on both you and your loved one.
- **Flooring and slip prevention:** Remove loose rugs or secure them with non-slip backing. Opt for slip-resistant flooring in high-risk areas such as the bathroom and kitchen.

A little foresight goes a long way. For example, imagine your loved one navigating a hallway scattered with shoes and bags – what seems like a small inconvenience to you could be a major hazard for them. Keeping pathways clear and ensuring proper lighting can help prevent unnecessary accidents.

2. **Leveraging Equipment and Assistive Devices**
   Assistive devices and home modifications can greatly improve mobility, safety and ease of care. The right equipment not only enhances your loved one's independence but also reduces physical strain on you as a caregiver, such as:

- **Mobility aids:** Consider walkers, rollators or wheelchairs suited to your loved one's needs. Adjustable-height chairs and beds can also help with mobility and transfers.
- **Ceiling hoists and lift systems:** If lifting and transferring your loved one is becoming physically demanding, ceiling hoists can make movement easier and safer.
- **Accessible bathrooms:** Install barrier-free showers, raised toilet seats and grab rails to ensure ease of use and prevent accidents.
- **Smart home technology:** Voice-activated lights, automated door openers and emergency alert systems can provide additional safety and convenience.

These tools can make daily care more manageable. For instance, a caregiver who struggled to help their mother transfer from bed to wheelchair found that installing a hoist system completely changed their experience, reducing back strain and increasing their mother's comfort.

Note: you may be eligible to access funds for equipment and modifications through the government funding programs discussed in Chapter 5, such as National Disability Insurance Scheme (NDIS) or Aged Care Packages.

3. **Maintaining a Clutter-Free and Organised Space**
   A well-organised home is not just about tidiness. It's about creating a safe and efficient space where everything has its place and is easily accessible when needed, like these:

   - **Designate storage areas for medical supplies and mobility aids:** Keep frequently used items within easy reach while ensuring they do not create hazards.

- **Label storage spaces:** Clearly labelled cupboards and drawers make it easier for caregivers and support workers to find essential items quickly.
- **Implement a regular decluttering routine:** Set aside time to assess and remove unnecessary items that could create hazards or clutter up key living spaces.
- **Pet management:** While pets provide companionship, they can also pose risks. Ensure they have a designated space during visits from support workers or when moving mobility aids.

Many caregivers find that once they create a dedicated space for essential items, daily tasks become smoother. For example, organising medical supplies in clearly marked containers means you won't have to scramble to find necessary items in an emergency.

4. **Responding to Injuries and Emergency Situations**
   Even with the best precautions, accidents can still happen. Being prepared ensures you can respond swiftly and effectively. Try these:

   - **First aid readiness:** Keep a well-stocked first aid kit in an accessible location and ensure you know how to use it.
   - **Emergency contact list:** Maintain a list of essential contacts, including medical professionals, family members and emergency services.
   - **Incident reporting and documentation:** If injuries occur, document them thoroughly to track patterns, identify risks and ensure appropriate follow-up care.
   - **Fire and evacuation plans:** Create and practice a simple emergency evacuation plan, ensuring that your loved one can exit the home safely if needed.

One caregiver recalled how their client, who used a walker, had a sudden fall in the bathroom. Because they had installed grab rails and kept an emergency response plan on hand, they were able to quickly assist the client and notify medical professionals without panic.

Action Steps:

- ✓ Conduct a home safety assessment using *WORKBOOK 7.13: Home Preparedness Checklist* and identify areas that need improvement
- ✓ Implement at least three changes this month, such as improving lighting, securing loose rugs or organising essential supplies
- ✓ Develop an emergency response plan with your family or support workers, following the guidance in *WORKBOOK 7.13: Emergency Response Plan and Incident Reporting*
- ✓ Ensure all support workers understand their responsibilities, including liability insurance and Occupational Health and Safety (OH&S) laws and document this in a service agreement

WORKBOOK 7.13: Home Preparation Checklist

Ensuring Security, Accessibility and Organisation

Use this checklist to assess your home environment and make necessary modifications to improve safety, accessibility and organisation.

☑ **General Home Safety**

- ☐ Fire extinguishers are accessible and regularly checked for functionality.
- ☐ A list of emergency phone numbers is displayed prominently for quick reference.
- ☐ All floors are free from clutter and tripping hazards (e.g. rugs, wires or furniture).
- ☐ Proper lighting is installed in hallways, staircases and main living areas.
- ☐ Motion-activated nightlights are placed in bedrooms, bathrooms and hallways.
- ☐ Smoke detectors are installed and tested regularly.

☑ **Accessibility Adjustments**

- ☐ Shower chairs and handheld showerheads are available for added convenience.
- ☐ Doorways and hallways are wide enough to accommodate wheelchairs and walkers.
- ☐ Grab rails are installed in key areas (e.g. bathroom, near the bed and along staircases).
- ☐ Non-slip mats are placed in the bathroom and kitchen to reduce fall risks.
- ☐ Ramps or stairlifts are available for individuals with mobility difficulties.
- ☐ Easy-to-use handles and knobs are installed on doors and cabinets.

✅ Organisation for Efficiency

- ☐ A weekly home maintenance checklist is in place to ensure ongoing safety improvements.
- ☐ A designated storage area is assigned for frequently used caregiving supplies.
- ☐ Important household documents, including insurance and medical records, are stored in a clearly labelled folder.
- ☐ Essential medical supplies are stored in an easily accessible location.
- ☐ Emergency contacts, including medical professionals and support workers, are listed and posted in a visible location.
- ☐ A dedicated area is set up for mobility aids, ensuring they are easy to access and use.
- ☐ Pets are safely contained during visits from support workers to prevent injuries.

✅ Safety Measures and Risk Management

- ☐ A service agreement is in place for all support workers, outlining responsibilities and expectations.
- ☐ Support workers have provided proof of liability and indemnity insurance.
- ☐ Occupational Health and Safety (OH&S) laws are reviewed and followed.
- ☐ A reporting system is in place for near misses, incidents and identified hazards.
- ☐ Support workers receive proper training in handling emergencies, including fire, medical and security threats.
- ☐ Fire exits and evacuation routes are clearly marked and accessible for all individuals, including those with mobility challenges.
- ☐ A protocol is in place to regularly inspect and maintain safety equipment, such as fire extinguishers, alarms and emergency lights.

WORKBOOK 7.13: Emergency Response Plan and Incident Report

Emergency Response Plan

Use this section to create a personalised emergency plan tailored to your home and caregiving situation.

Emergency Contacts
☐ Family Member/s: _________________ Phone: _____________
☐ Doctor/Healthcare Provider: __________ Phone: _________
☐ Nearest Hospital: _______________ Phone: _____________
☐ Local Emergency Services: __________ Phone: _________
☐ Support Workers/Agency: __________ Phone: _________

Emergency Response Procedures
☐ Assess the situation and determine the appropriate response (evacuation, shelter-in-place or medical assistance).
☐ Assign roles and responsibilities to household members or support workers in case of an emergency.
☐ Establish clear communication methods to alert emergency services and family members if needed.
☐ Conduct regular emergency drills, including fire, medical and security response scenarios.

First Aid Preparedness
☐ A fully stocked first aid kit is easily accessible.
☐ Medications are labelled and stored properly.
☐ A CPR and first aid guide is available and reviewed periodically.
☐ Support workers are trained in emergency response procedures.

Incident Report Form
Use this form to document any accidents or incidents that occur
in the home.

Date of Incident: _______________________________________
Time of Incident: _______________________________________
Location: ____
Individuals Involved:

____

Description of Incident:

____

____

____

Immediate Actions Taken:

____

____

____

Was Emergency Services Contacted? ☐ Yes ☐ No

Additional Notes:

____

____

____

Completed By: _____________________ **Date:** _______________

As a result of this incident/accident, are there any follow-up reviews
necessary? Any documents to be updated? ☐ Yes ☐ No

Notes:

____

____

PART 3:
THE FINAL PIECE

Adapting, Communicating and Moving Forward

Caregiving is never static – it evolves with time, circumstances and the changing needs of your loved one. This final section brings everything together, helping you navigate the transitions ahead with confidence and clarity.

We'll explore how to communicate effectively, maintain safety and anticipate future needs so you can adapt with ease. You'll also reflect on where you are now and what's next, ensuring you have the tools and mindset to continue this journey with strength and purpose.

While caregiving may shift and change, one thing remains constant – you are not alone in this. Let's take the next step together.

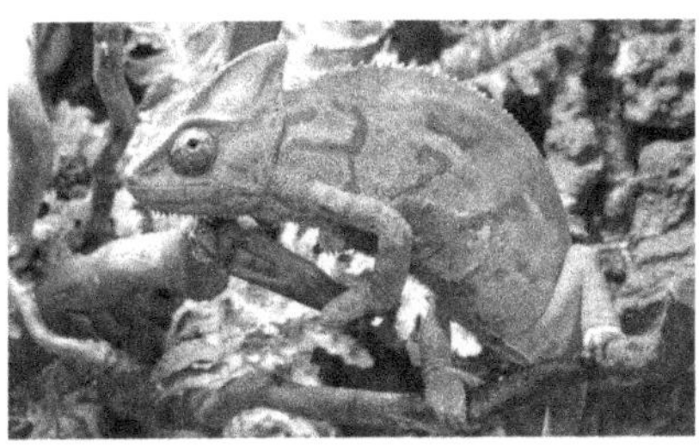

"With experience, the chameleon no longer reacts – it anticipates. It knows when to stand out, when to blend in and how to navigate the ever-changing world with confidence and wisdom." (Andrea Entwistle)

CHAPTER 8

The Power of Connection

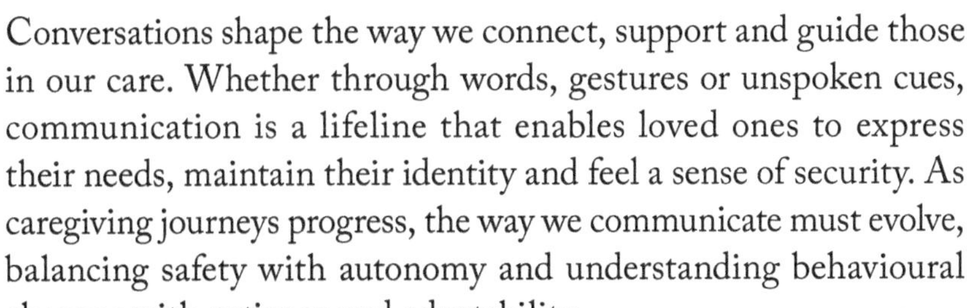

Conversations shape the way we connect, support and guide those in our care. Whether through words, gestures or unspoken cues, communication is a lifeline that enables loved ones to express their needs, maintain their identity and feel a sense of security. As caregiving journeys progress, the way we communicate must evolve, balancing safety with autonomy and understanding behavioural changes with patience and adaptability.

This chapter will focus on the critical role of effective communication in caregiving, particularly when a loved one's needs change due to illness, ageing or cognitive decline. We will explore how to identify and respond to behavioural changes, adapt communication strategies to meet evolving needs and maintain a respectful dialogue that prioritises both safety and autonomy.

Additionally, we will discuss methods to ensure integrational safety while preserving a loved one's sense of control and dignity. This chapter will offer practical guidance on overcoming resistance to support, adapting to changes in speech and understanding and finding new ways to stay connected with your loved one. With clear strategies, you can navigate these challenges while maintaining confidence and care.

A crucial part of communication in caregiving is knowing when and how to discuss future care needs. As a loved one's condition progresses, there may come a time when staying at home is no longer the safest or most feasible option. This chapter will also explore the importance of early conversations about future needs, including when to discuss the possibility of transitioning to a care facility. Approaching these discussions with sensitivity, respect and an open mind can help ensure that decisions are made collaboratively rather than in crisis situations.

Effective communication is the foundation of caregiving, helping to reduce stress, maintain trust and ensure the well-being of your loved one. By understanding how communication shapes their experience, you can adapt to their needs while preserving their sense of dignity and autonomy.

Why is Communication So Important?

Clear communication reduces anxiety by addressing confusion, frustration or fear that may arise due to changes in health or ability. When caregivers communicate calmly and clearly, it helps build trust and ease emotional distress, making daily interactions smoother and more reassuring.

Supporting decision-making empowers loved ones by giving them a voice in their care. Even small choices, such as selecting meals or choosing activities, help maintain independence and self-esteem.

When caregivers facilitate discussions about preferences and concerns, they reinforce a sense of control rather than taking it away.

Respectful dialogue strengthens relationships by fostering connection and understanding. Open conversations encourage your loved one to express their thoughts, feelings and concerns. This builds a deeper bond and makes them feel valued, ensuring that they remain engaged in their own care journey rather than feeling like a passive recipient of assistance.

Adapting communication enhances safety by recognising when a loved one struggles with comprehension or speech. If verbal instructions become difficult, using visual cues, written prompts or non-verbal gestures can prevent misunderstandings and reduce risks. Adjusting how you communicate ensures that they remain and feel as safe and independent as possible.

Feeling heard supports emotional well-being by reducing stress, frustration and emotional withdrawal. When caregivers take the time to listen, acknowledge concerns and validate emotions, it reassures loved ones that their thoughts and feelings matter. This strengthens their confidence and overall quality of life.

"Communication works for those who work at it."
(John Powell)

Understanding Key Terms

- *Integrational Safety* – The balance between independence and protection, ensuring a loved one's safety while allowing them the dignity of choice.
- *Behavioural Adaptation* – The process of adjusting responses and strategies to match a loved one's evolving needs and reactions.

- *Freedom of Choice in Care* – Recognising and respecting a loved one's autonomy in decision-making while guiding them toward safe and practical choices.

As a loved one's condition changes, communication and support must also evolve to meet new challenges. Adjusting to their needs ensures they feel understood, respected and secure. This section explores three critical areas that can help caregivers respond effectively:

- Recognising behavioural changes
- Balancing safety with autonomy
- Modifying communication methods to maintain connection

Let's look at these three topics in more depth and expand on each one of them.

1. Recognising Behavioural Changes

Behaviour can stem from cognitive decline, emotional distress, physical discomfort or an underlying condition that has been present since birth. Some individuals may struggle to communicate clearly, understand social cues or manage overwhelming external environments due to conditions such as autism, intellectual disabilities or neurological disorders. These challenges can lead to frustration, withdrawal or behavioural outbursts, making effective communication even more vital.

Seeking professional assessment and advice is essential in identifying the root cause of these behavioural changes. A formal diagnosis can provide clarity and offer tailored communication strategies to better support you and your loved one. Health professionals, speech therapists and behavioural specialists can help caregivers understand and implement appropriate techniques to improve interaction and reduce stress.

By taking proactive steps, you can ensure that communication remains supportive, respectful and adapted to your loved one's unique needs. Recognising the triggers can help prevent conflict and distress. Common triggers may include changes in routine, sensory overload, miscommunication or unmet needs.

Being aware of these potential stressors allows caregivers to proactively adjust the environment and approach situations with patience and understanding. Developing strategies to handle these challenges, such as providing clear instructions, using visual schedules or allowing extra processing time, can significantly improve interactions.

Additionally, ensuring that other support people – such as family members, friends or professional carers – are informed about your loved one's communication preferences and triggers can enhance the quality of care. Sharing strategies and insights with those involved in their daily life will not only make caregiving more consistent but also create a respectful and accommodating environment in the community.

This collaborative effort ensures that your loved one is treated with dignity and provided with the right support in a way that works best for them. Consider a scenario where your loved one becomes increasingly withdrawn or resistant to routine care. Instead of enforcing rigid expectations, approach them with gentle questioning: 'I've noticed you seem a little quieter today. Would you like to talk about what's on your mind?'

A non-confrontational approach fosters trust and encourages openness.

2. Respecting Freedom of Choice While Ensuring Safety

Autonomy is a fundamental human right and respecting your loved one's choices is crucial in maintaining their dignity and independence. However, there are times when their decisions may pose a risk to their health or safety and as a caregiver, you have a duty of care to ensure their well-being. While honouring their preferences is essential, there are situations where intervention is necessary.

For example, a person with diabetes may crave sugary foods like cake or lollies and attempt to obtain them when you are not home. They may use the opportunity to ask another family member or support worker for these items, potentially putting their health at risk. In such cases, clear communication is essential to ensure that everyone involved in their care understands the boundaries and responsibilities required to keep them safe.

Establishing strategies and protocols for handling these situations is key. Caregivers should communicate with all support persons – including family members, friends and professional carers – to ensure consistency in care. This can include setting firm yet respectful guidelines, offering suitable alternatives and using gentle redirection techniques. It is not about denying their choices but guiding them toward safer decisions that prioritise their well-being.

Encouraging open discussions with your loved one about their health and safety can also help them understand these pose importance of these measures for you. Phrasing concerns in a supportive rather than restrictive manner, such as, 'I know you enjoy sweets and I want to find a way for you to have something you like while keeping your health in check,' can make the conversation more collaborative rather than confrontational.

By fostering a shared understanding of boundaries and safe choices, caregivers can respect autonomy while still upholding their responsibility to provide protection and care. Suppose your loved one insists on cooking despite declining mobility. Instead of outright refusal, present safer alternatives: 'I love that you still want to cook. How about we prep the ingredients together and I help with the hot surfaces?' This approach validates their desire for independence while subtly reducing risks.

3. Adapting to Evolving Communication Needs

As conditions progress, your loved one may face increasing challenges in speech, comprehension and expression. This decline is common in conditions such as Multiple Sclerosis (MS), where cognitive function remains intact but verbal communication becomes difficult. In such cases, adaptive communication tools are vital to helping them express their needs clearly.

Assistive technology, such as speech-generating devices, text-tospeech apps and tools like *Neuronode*, which can be controlled through visual or physical movement, can greatly enhance their ability to communicate eff ectively. Th ese tools enable them to make calls, control household devices or engage in conversations with minimal frustration.

In contrast, cognitive conditions such as Alzheimer's disease impact comprehension, memory retention and the ability to process information. This often results in repetitive questions, confusion with daily tasks or a tendency to recall past events while struggling with short-term memory. In these situations, communication strategies should focus on simplifying language, maintaining patience and using familiar cues. Visual aids, such as placing pictures of support workers near the door to help them recognise visitors, can aid in reducing anxiety and resistance.

Active listening, clear verbal cues and non-patronising redirection techniques are essential for maintaining meaningful communication as conditions deteriorate. Simplifying language without being condescending and reinforcing important information through repetition can help prevent frustration and strengthen understanding.

It is also important to involve healthcare and allied health professionals in assessing and reassessing communication needs. Speech therapists, occupational therapists and assistive technology specialists can recommend tools and strategies that align with your loved one's evolving requirements. Many of these services and devices may be eligible through *NDIS* funding, ensuring that your loved one receives the necessary support to maintain their communication abilities and quality of life.

4. Having Early Conversations About Future Needs

One of the most difficult conversations in caregiving is discussing the possibility of moving into a care facility. Most loved ones do not want to hear about it until there is no other option. However, in some circumstances, it is necessary to have this conversation early, particularly for those with cognitive and degenerative conditions while they are still of sound mind. This allows them to express their wishes about where they would like to live in the future and ensures their preferences are respected.

Caregivers often express concerns about this topic, as delaying the discussion can lead to stress and uncertainty. Without a plan in place, the conversation often becomes rushed and emotionally charged when a crisis arises. When decisions cannot be made collaboratively, it can create frustration and guilt for both the caregiver and their loved one.

Another common challenge is the outright refusal to address the topic at all. When the conversation is avoided entirely, it can leave families unprepared when their loved one can no longer remain at home safely. In these instances, it is helpful to take a gradual approach – slowly introducing the idea, planting the seed over time and reassuring them that planning does not mean an immediate change. Simple phrases like 'I just want to have a plan in place, not because you need it now but because it gives me peace of mind that you can make the choice while you are able to' can help ease resistance.

Reassuring your loved one that the priority is to keep them at home for as long as possible, while having a contingency plan, can create a sense of security. Good communication ensures that everyone involved is on the same page, reducing anxiety and fostering a more positive and proactive approach to future care planning. Many caregivers avoid this topic until a crisis arises, making the transition more stressful. Here are some tips for approaching this conversation early:

- **Start Gradually**: Introduce the topic casually before it becomes an urgent necessity. Mentioning examples from friends or family can make it feel less personal and confrontational.
- **Acknowledge Their Feelings**: Reassure your loved one that their preferences and fears matter. Phrases like 'I know this is a difficult subject but I want us to be prepared together' can help open up the discussion.
- **Present Options, Not Ultimatums**: Rather than saying 'You need to move into a care home,' *consider* 'Let's explore different support options so you can remain comfortable and safe.'
- **Involve Professionals**: Seeking advice from doctors, social workers or aged care advisors can provide additional guidance and credibility.

Addressing common concerns is an important part of caregiving, as many challenges arise when balancing a loved one's needs, independence and overall well-being. Understanding these concerns and having strategies in place can help ensure smoother interactions and better outcomes for both caregivers and those receiving care.

You may feel that certain conversations are too complex or uncomfortable to approach – let's explore some common concerns and how to navigate them with confidence.

'My loved one refuses to use mobility aids or accept assistance. How do I encourage them without making them feel helpless?'
Instead of framing it as a loss of independence, highlight the benefits: 'This will help you move around more easily and continue doing the things you enjoy.' Encouragement over enforcement is key.

'What if my loved one becomes aggressive or uncooperative?'
Behavioural changes often stem from frustration or fear. Stay calm, identify potential triggers and use distraction or redirection to ease tension. If the behaviour persists, consider professional advice to rule out underlying health issues.

'I struggle to keep track of changes in my loved one's behaviour and communication. How can I make this process easier?'
Using a Care Communication Log can be a helpful tool in tracking changes, identifying patterns and ensuring that all support workers are informed about evolving needs. Documenting daily interactions, mood changes and communication challenges allows for better coordination and proactive adjustments in care. It also provides valuable insights for discussions with healthcare professionals, helping to tailor support strategies effectively. There is a Care Communication Log at the end of this chapter for you to use.

Take Action

- ✓ Now that you have explored the importance of effective communication and the strategies to support your loved one, it's time to put these insights into action.
- ✓ Initiate early conversations about future care needs – use *WORKBOOK 8: Approaching and Assessing Communication Needs*
- ✓ Maintain a Care Communication Log using *WORKBOOK 8: Care Communication Log*
- ✓ Ensure Continuity Among Support Workers

WORKBOOK 8: Approaching and Assessing Communication Needs

✅ Step 1: Assessing Communication Needs

Before having a conversation, it's important to recognise how your loved one processes and expresses information. Use this checklist to assess their communication style and potential barriers:

Understanding Their Communication Ability:
- ☐ Can they express their needs clearly?
- ☐ Do they struggle with verbal communication?
- ☐ Have there been recent changes in how they communicate?
- ☐ Are they comfortable using assistive communication tools (e.g., speech devices, writing aids)?

Recognising Emotional and Cognitive Barriers:
- ☐ Do they become frustrated or withdrawn during conversations?
- ☐ Are they experiencing cognitive decline, making it harder to follow discussions?
- ☐ Are they resistant to discussing certain topics (e.g., future care, mobility aids)?

Identifying Environmental and Situational Challenges:
- ☐ Are there distractions (TV, noise) that make communication difficult?
- ☐ Are they more receptive to discussions at specific times of the day?
- ☐ Do they need extra time to process and respond?

Action: Identify one key communication challenge you want to address and write it here:

____

____

____

____

✅ Step 2: Preparing for Difficult Conversations

Difficult conversations require planning. Whether you need to discuss safety concerns, evolving care needs or future plans, use this framework to prepare:

Clarify Your Goal:
- ☐ What do you need to communicate?
- ☐ What outcome do you hope for?
- ☐ How can you phrase your message with care and respect?

Consider Their Perspective:
- ☐ What concerns might they have?
- ☐ How might they react?
- ☐ How can you acknowledge their feelings while guiding the conversation?

Choose the Right Setting:
- ☐ Find a quiet, comfortable space
- ☐ Ensure enough time for discussion without rushing
- ☐ Minimise distractions and interruptions

Action: Write a short opening statement for your conversation: *'I want to talk about [topic] because I care about your well-being and want to find the best way forward together.'*

☑ Step 3: Approaching the Conversation with Care

Use these conversation techniques to create a safe and respectful dialogue:

1. Start with Empathy:
- ☐ Acknowledge their feelings: 'I know this might be difficult to talk about but I want to understand what's important to you.'
- ☐ Show that you are listening with open body language and patience.

2. Use Gentle Encouragement:
- ☐ Instead of saying, 'You need to stop doing that,' try, 'I want to make sure you stay safe – can we find a way that works for both of us?'
- ☐ Offer alternatives instead of ultimatums: 'Would you feel more comfortable if we explored some options together?'

3. Stay Calm and Redirect If Needed:
- ☐ If they become defensive, take a step back and reassure them: 'We don't have to decide today but I want to keep the conversation open.'
- ☐ If the discussion becomes emotional, suggest a break and return to it later.

Action: Write one supportive phrase you can use during the conversation:

____

____

____

____

____

____

____

☑ Step 4: Following Up and Adjusting Your Approach

Conversations about care and safety are ongoing. Use this checklist to reflect and adjust as needed:

- ☐ Did your loved one feel heard?
- ☐ Were you able to find common ground?
- ☐ Do you need to revisit the conversation at a later time?
- ☐ Are there professionals (speech therapists, social workers) who can help?

Action: Note one thing you learned from the conversation and how you can improve next time:

____

____

____

____

WORKBOOK 8: Care Communication Log

Purpose of the Log:

- To monitor changes in communication abilities, behaviour and comprehension.
- To ensure continuity of care among support workers and family members.
- To provide documented insights for health professionals, aiding in assessments and treatment planning.

How to Use This Log:

- Record entries daily or after significant interactions.
- Be objective and specific in noting observations.
- Use the log to reflect on patterns, challenges and successes

Daily Communication Log Template

Date	Time	Support Worker	Observations and Interactions	Changes in Communication	Actions Taken	Notes for Next Support Worker

Instructions:

- **Observations and Interactions:** Note any significant conversations, interactions or emotional responses.
- **Changes in Communication:** Identify shifts in verbal abilities, comprehension or non-verbal cues.
- **Actions Taken:** Describe any responses or strategies used to assist communication.
- **Notes for Next Support Worker:** Provide insights or recommendations for the next shift.

Weekly Summary and Reflection

1. Key Changes Noted This Week:

- _______________________________________
- _______________________________________
- _______________________________________

2. Challenges Encountered and Strategies Used:

- ____
- ____
- ____

3. Recommendations for Improvement:

- ____
- ____
- ____

Emergency and Crisis Communication Plan

Recognising Signs of Distress:
- Sudden withdrawal or refusal to communicate.
- Increased agitation or signs of frustration.
- Difficulty understanding or processing information.

Immediate Steps to Take:
- Stay calm and use reassuring body language.
- Remove unnecessary distractions and create a quiet environment.
- Use simple phrases, visual aids or non-verbal gestures to assist understanding.

Who to Contact in Case of Emergency:

Name: ____

Relationship: ____________________________________

Contact Number: _________________________________

Preferred Medical Professional: _______________________

CHAPTER 9

Shaping What's Next: Your Roadmap

As you turn the final pages of this book, take a deep breath and acknowledge how far you've come. Caregiving is not a role we prepare for – it's a journey that unfolds, full of challenges, learning curves and moments of deep love. You have walked this path with dedication and that alone is something to be proud of.

Caregiving is a journey that cannot be contained within a single book, no matter how comprehensive. There will always be moments when you feel lost, when questions arise and when new challenges demand more than words on a page can provide. The good news? You are not alone. This is not the end. Rather, it is an invitation to continue growing, learning and building a caregiving system that supports you and your loved ones fully.

You don't have to figure everything out on your own. There are tangible, real-world ways to continue this journey with expert support, community and transformative tools designed just for you.

> *"Alone we can do so little; together we can do so much."*
> (Helen Keller)

Why Reflection and Next Steps Matter

1. **Acknowledging Growth Builds Confidence**
   Looking back at how far you've come is just as important as looking ahead. Every small step – whether learning a new approach, creating a system or simply recognising when you need help – adds up to something bigger. Caregiving is a journey of constant adaptation and acknowledging your progress helps build the confidence to continue moving forward.

2. **Caregiving Is Ever-Changing – As Should Be Your Approach**
   What worked six months ago may not work now and that's okay. The needs of your loved one, your personal boundaries and even your available resources will shift over time. Embracing continuous learning and flexibility ensures you stay prepared and resilient.

3. **Support Networks Make the Journey Easier**
   Caregiving often feels isolating but you don't have to do it alone. Seeking support – whether from professional guidance, peer networks or structured learning – reduces stress and makes the journey more sustainable. Studies show that caregivers who actively engage in support groups or training experience significantly lower burnout rates.

4. **Emotional and Mental Well-Being Are Essential**
   It's easy to prioritise the needs of your loved one over your own but neglecting your well-being leads to exhaustion and resentment. You cannot pour from an empty cup – taking care of yourself ensures that you can continue to provide care without losing yourself in the process.

What This Chapter Covers

This chapter will help you:

- Reflect on your caregiving journey and acknowledge your progress
- Understand the importance of continuous learning and support
- Identify what's next for you and how to move forward with clarity
- Explore how support networks can sustain and uplift you
- Prepare for the next steps with practical action steps

By the end of this chapter, you will have a clear understanding of how to transition from learning to implementation, ensuring that caregiving remains sustainable and fulfilling for both you and your loved one.

How to Move Forward with Confidence

Now that you have reflected on your journey and identified what you need next, let's explore practical ways to move forward. Caregiving doesn't have to feel overwhelming – small, intentional changes can create lasting improvements.

Each step below is paired with real-life examples to illustrate how you can integrate these insights into your caregiving journey. Additionally, *WORKBOOK 9: Reflecting and Moving Forward* provides guided activities to help you process each step, reflect on your progress and create a clear plan for the road ahead.

1. Take a Moment to Reflect

Before planning the next steps, take time to acknowledge what you've gained from this journey. Reflection brings clarity – it allows you to see what's working, what's not and where you need support.

Maria's Lightbulb Moment:

Maria, one of my coaching clients, had been caring for her father with Parkinson's for two years. She was exhausted, constantly second-guessing her decisions and felt like she wasn't doing enough. As part of our work together, we focused on shifting her perspective by identifying the progress she had already made.

Together, we explored how her caregiving had evolved – how she had learned to communicate better, set up a medication schedule and create small moments of joy for her father. When she finally put these reflections on paper, she saw her growth in a new light. This process helped her realise she wasn't failing; she was adapting.

2. Define What You Need Next

Once you've reflected, the next step is identifying what kind of support will help you move forward. Caregiving isn't one-size-fits-all – your next step should be tailored to what you need most right now. Gaining clarity on your needs allows you to make informed decisions and avoid unnecessary stress.

James Learns to Ask for Help:

James, one of my coaching clients, was balancing full-time work while caring for his mother with early-stage dementia. He was convinced he had to handle everything alone until he realised he was constantly overwhelmed and struggling to keep up. In our sessions, we worked on defining what would make caregiving more sustainable for him.

Together, we identified three areas that needed the most attention – structuring his daily routine, building a support network and creating dedicated time for self-care.

Through this process, James saw that asking for help wasn't a sign of weakness but a strategy for long-term success. With a clearer direction, he was able to take practical steps toward easing his caregiving load, knowing he didn't have to do it all alone.

3. Build a Plan for Continued Support

Caregiving is more sustainable when you have a plan. This doesn't mean creating a rigid structure – it means developing a framework that supports both you and your loved one in a way that feels manageable. Whether it's refining caregiving systems, connecting with a support network or setting boundaries to protect your well-being, having a plan in place reduces stress and brings clarity to daily challenges.

A Caregiver's 'What If' Plan:

Another client of mine was caring for her two grown sons with disabilities. She carried the weight of responsibility every day, constantly worrying about what would happen if she became unable to care for them, even temporarily. Together, we worked on creating a care plan binder – a structured but simple system where she could document essential information, including medical schedules, emergency contacts and daily routines.

Through this process, she realised she had been holding onto all the information in her head, which made her anxiety even greater. By putting it into a structured format, she felt a sense of relief, knowing that if something unexpected happened, there was a clear guide for others to step in. She also arranged for regular respite care, giving herself consistent time to rest and recharge. Having this plan in place didn't just provide practical support – it gave her peace of mind, knowing her sons would always have the care they needed.

4. Strengthen Emotional Resilience

Caregiving is more than just logistics – it's deeply emotional. Moments of frustration, guilt and exhaustion are natural but long-term resilience comes from recognising these feelings, processing them and finding ways to protect your own well-being. When you give yourself permission to acknowledge your emotions, you create space for balance and strength in your caregiving role.

My Breaking Point as a Caregiver:

There was a time in my own caregiving journey when I felt completely depleted. I was juggling responsibilities, doing everything I could to provide care but inside, I was running on empty. One day, after a particularly difficult moment, I found myself on the verge of tears over something small – not because of what had happened in that moment but because of the weight of everything I had been carrying. I had been so focused on managing everything that I didn't allow myself to process the emotional toll.

I knew something had to change. I started to prioritise small but meaningful moments of self-care, from journaling my thoughts to seeking out others who truly understood the challenges I was facing. Eventually, I connected with a support network where I could talk openly, share experiences and feel seen. That shift didn't take away the challenges but it made them feel less isolating. I learned that asking for support wasn't a weakness – it was a way to sustain both myself and my ability to care for others.

5. Take Action – One Step at a Time

Caregiving can feel overwhelming when you try to fix everything at once. The key to making real progress is focusing on small, intentional steps that create meaningful change. By tackling one thing at a time, you build a more sustainable approach to caregiving – one that allows you to manage responsibilities while also taking care of yourself.

Karen's Journey to Stability:

Karen, one of my coaching clients, was juggling the responsibilities of being a mother and wife while managing a debilitating back condition. As the demands of her life grew, she found herself struggling to keep up with household tasks, self-care and emotional well-being. She felt like everything was spiralling, unsure of where to even begin regaining control.

Together, we focused on small, structured changes that would create a lasting impact. We established essential household systems, ensuring there were clear written instructions so others could step in and support her when needed. Weekly coaching sessions provided her with both accountability and encouragement as she worked toward her health and emotional goals.

By breaking things down into manageable steps, Karen not only regained stability in her life but also created space to prioritise her well-being without guilt. She discovered that real change doesn't happen overnight but with consistent, small steps, she could move forward with clarity, confidence and the support she needed.

To take these insights a step further, go to *WORKBOOK 9: Reflecting and Moving Forward* and work through the exercises designed to help you map out your next steps. This will give you the space to organise your thoughts, identify key areas for improvement and create a plan that makes your caregiving journey more structured and manageable. By taking the time to reflect and put things into action, you can move forward with greater clarity and confidence.

You may have doubts about whether reflecting, planning or seeking support will truly make a difference. Here are some common concerns caregivers often have, along with ways to shift perspective and make caregiving more manageable.

'I don't have time to sit down and reflect – I'm already stretched too thin.'
Taking a few moments to reflect and plan now can actually save you time in the long run. The workbook is designed to be simple and effective, helping you identify small changes that can make caregiving more manageable. Even setting aside just five minutes can give you clarity and ease some of the mental load.

'I should be able to handle this on my own – asking for help feels like I'm failing.'
Seeking support isn't a sign of failure; it's a strategy for long-term success. Caregiving is a demanding role and no one is meant to do it alone. Having a plan, a support network and structured guidance allows you to be a better caregiver while also looking after your own well-being.

'I don't see how a workbook or planning will change anything – my situation is just too overwhelming.'
Feeling overwhelmed is completely understandable but having a structured approach can help you regain control, even in small ways. The workbook isn't about adding more to your plate – it's about simplifying your role and giving you tools to lighten the load. Every step, no matter how small, moves you toward a more balanced caregiving experience.

Take Action

- ✓ Go through *WORKBOOK 9: Reflecting and Moving Forward*
- ✓ Identify one small, actionable change you can make today
- ✓ Commit to ongoing support and learning

WORKBOOK 9: Reflecting and Moving Forward

Taking Action for a More Sustainable and Balanced Caregiving Journey

This workbook is designed to help you take practical, manageable steps toward improving your caregiving experience. By working through the sections below, you'll gain clarity on where you are now, what you need next and how to create a plan for moving forward with confidence.

☑ Step 1: Acknowledge How Far You've Come
- Set aside 10 minutes today to reflect on your caregiving journey.
- Write down three lessons you've learned and how they've helped you grow.
- Identify one challenge you need support with and make a plan to address it.

Reflection Prompts:

What has been the most valuable lesson you've learned from this book?

____

What small change have you made that has made caregiving easier?

____

What challenge do you still struggle with?

____

☑ Step 2: Define What You Need Next
- Identify one caregiving area that needs improvement (e.g., daily structure, emotional support, self-care).

- Research one resource or support option that aligns with your need (e.g., caregiver groups, training, respite services, coaching).
- Write down one action you can take this week to move toward a solution.

Reflection Prompts:

What is one thing that, if improved, would make caregiving feel easier?

____

Who or what could help you with this? (e.g., professional support, tools, resources)

____

What is one action you can take today to move toward a solution?

____

✅ Step 3: Build a Plan for Continued Support

- Create or refine a caregiving system – start with something simple like a shared calendar for appointments.
- Find one new support system – whether that's a friend, caregiver group or professional guidance.
- Schedule self-care – even if it's just 30 minutes a week focused on yourself.

Reflection Prompts:

What is one system you can create or improve to make caregiving easier?

____

Who is one person or group you can turn to for support?

____

What is one way you can prioritise your own well-being this week?

____

☑ Step 4: Strengthen Emotional Resilience

- Recognise emotional triggers – identify what situations cause stress or guilt for you.
- Find a safe space – whether that's a support group, therapist or friend.
- Allow yourself to step back – taking a break isn't neglecting care; it's ensuring you can keep going.

Reflection Prompts:

What emotions come up most often in your caregiving role (e.g., stress, guilt, frustration)?

____

Who can you talk to when you need emotional support?

____

What is one way you can take a break or decompress this week?

____

☑ Step 5: Take Action – One Step at a Time

- Pick ONE caregiving challenge and commit to improving it this week.
- Break it down into small steps – what's the first action you can take?
- Track progress – at the end of the week, reflect: Did this change help? What's next?

Reflection Prompts:

What caregiving challenge will you focus on this week?

____

What is the first action you can take toward improving this?

____

At the end of the week, how did it go? Did it help?

____

Afterword

Congratulations! You have not only reached the final pages of this book but have also embraced the essence of what it means to be adaptable, resilient and ever-evolving – just like the chameleon.

At the start of this journey, you were like the young chameleon, stepping into unfamiliar territory and learning how to navigate the challenges of caregiving. Along the way, you developed systems, synchronised routines and built the confidence to adapt – mirroring the teenage chameleon learning to blend with its surroundings.

And now, as you reach this final chapter, you have grown into the wise, mature chameleon – aware of the landscape, prepared for changes and confident in your ability to adapt while protecting your own well-being.

Caregiving, like the chameleon's journey, is about flexibility, resilience and finding balance in ever-changing circumstances. It's about learning when to blend in and when to stand out, when to hold steady and when to move forward. No matter what lies ahead, you now have the tools, the awareness and the support to navigate it with confidence.

This is not the end of your journey – it's a transformation. You have become the chameleon, capable of adapting, growing and thriving. Embrace this new chapter with the wisdom and strength you have gained, knowing that you are never alone.

It has been an absolute privilege to guide you on this journey. I know that the road of caregiving is often filled with uncertainty, exhaustion and deep emotional moments – both joyful and challenging. If you've made it to the end of this book, it means you've not only sought answers but have also been willing to reflect, grow and commit to making a difference in your own life and in the life of your loved one. That is something truly worth celebrating!

If there's anything in this book that sparked a question, a thought or even a new perspective, I would love to hear from you. Caregiving is never a journey meant to be walked alone and I want you to know that I am here.

Your experiences, your challenges and your victories matter. Every caregiver's journey is different – some days you might feel strong and capable and others might leave you feeling completely overwhelmed. I understand this because I have been there, too. I know what it's like to stand in the middle of a difficult moment, feeling as though no one could possibly understand the weight of your responsibilities. But I also know the power of connection – the way a single conversation, a shared story or a new perspective can completely change the way you experience caregiving.

That's why I want to encourage you to reach out, to share your thoughts and to ask questions. Whether you need clarity on something discussed in these pages or you simply want to reflect on how this book has supported you, I would love to hear from you.

More than anything, I want you to know that your voice matters. So often, caregivers become invisible, lost in the needs of those they care for. It's easy to forget that you, too, are a person with needs, dreams and a life outside of your caregiving role.

If there is anything I hope you take away from this book, it is that your well-being is just as important as the well-being of your loved one. You deserve support, encouragement and guidance just as much as they do. And if you ever feel like you are alone, please know that you are not. There is an entire community of caregivers – people just like you – who are walking this path and who understand the emotions, the sacrifices and the love that comes with it.

You are part of something much larger than just your day-to-day responsibilities and you are never alone in this journey.

If you ever feel uncertain, if you ever question whether you're doing enough or if you simply want to connect with someone who truly understands, I am here. Supporting caregivers is not just what I do – it is my mission, my passion and my purpose. And if this book has helped you in any way, if it has given you even a small piece of hope or a new way of looking at your caregiving journey, then it has served its purpose.

Never hesitate to reach out, because I would love nothing more than to continue supporting you in any way I can.

I would love to hear your story. How has this book supported you? What changes have you made, even in small ways, that have helped you feel more empowered as a caregiver? When I was caring for my mum, I longed for a book like this – something that could have guided me through the complexities of caregiving while also reminding me not to forget myself in the process.

If this book has given you even a fraction of the guidance and encouragement I wished for during my own journey, then that is the greatest gift I could ever receive.

My 'why' – the reason I do this work – is to inspire caregivers who feel lost, exhausted or overwhelmed. I know the frustration, the grief and the deep sense of responsibility that can sometimes feel all-consuming. But I also know that there is hope. There are answers. And most importantly, there are others – people like you – who are walking this same path. You are not alone. Caregivers across the world deserve to feel strong, confident and supported.

My dream is to see caregivers everywhere standing tall, embracing self-care without guilt and knowing that they are just as important as the loved ones they care for.

Through structured systems, well-designed programs and a community of support, we can redefine what caregiving looks like. We can make it a journey of connection rather than depletion, of joy rather than just duty.

At some stage or another, we all need a voice – we need to be heard, understood and uplifted. And that is what I hope this book has done for you.

So, once again, congratulations on completing this book. This is not the end of your caregiving journey but rather the beginning of a new, more sustainable and fulfilling chapter.

This is your first step towards a caregiving experience that not only serves your loved one but also honours your own well-being. I trust that one day our paths will cross and when they do, I hope to call you a friend.

Take care of yourself – you deserve it. And never forget that you are doing an incredible job. Congratulations!

With love and gratitude,
Andrea

Get in touch with me:
Website: *https://a1-quality-care.com*
Email: *admin@a1-quality-care.com*

About The Author

Andrea Entwistle is a coach, author and lifelong caregiver, dedicated to empowering those navigating the complexities of caregiving. She is the founder of *A1 Quality Care*, where she provides support, resilience-building and systems to help caregivers find balance in their demanding roles.

Originally from the Czech Republic, Andrea was raised in a family of carers – her father an anaesthetist, her mother a nurse – where the values of compassion and service were deeply ingrained in her from a young age. With over 20 years in the disability industry, she has worked across management, quality and compliance, later transitioning into projects and consulting to identify and bridge gaps in management systems.

Despite her corporate success, she felt a deep need to return to hands-on caregiving – where real impact happens. Becoming a support worker and coach was a pivotal moment, bringing her back to the heart of care.

Her most defining and life-altering experience came when her mother was diagnosed with cancer. Stepping into the role of a caregiver on an intensely personal level, Andrea walked the heartbreaking journey of seeing a vibrant, independent woman slowly become fragile. Knowing that survival was not an option, she grieved alongside her mother while juggling work, family and the emotional weight of impending loss. Through that pain, she found her purpose: to create *A1 Quality Care*, offering caregivers the guidance, systems and coaching they so desperately need.

A lifelong learner, Andrea holds qualifications in business management, quality, risk and compliance, coaching, training and assessment, hypnotherapy and nutrition. She is now deepening her studies in counselling, further enriching her ability to guide and empower others.

Andrea lives on the Bellarine Peninsula in Ocean Grove, Australia – a place of breathtaking beauty that nourishes her soul. Whether she's surfing, walking along the shore, swimming or spending time with her beloved dogs, the ocean is her sanctuary. A mother of three and a proud grandmother to two granddaughters, she finds endless joy in the richness of family life. Her husband, whom she calls her rock in life, has been a constant source of love, support and unwavering encouragement, standing beside her through every challenge and triumph.

Fluent in five languages, Andrea embraces cultures, travel and personal growth, believing that exploring the world is one of the greatest educations she can offer her children. She has travelled extensively and plans to continue doing so, knowing that real-world experiences offer the best lessons in adaptability, understanding and appreciation for diversity. Travel, for her, is not just an adventure but a way to instil lifelong curiosity and wisdom in her children.

Deeply spiritual, she finds solace in meditation, breathwork and yoga, balancing her innate drive with moments of reflection and peace. She has an undeniable love for humour – though she admits she's hopeless at telling jokes, she never fails to appreciate a good one.

Her father remains a guiding force in her life, a well of wisdom and encouragement. While the loss of her mother left an irreplaceable void, Andrea feels her presence in every step of her journey, driving her mission forward. *A1 Quality Care* is not just a business – it is the embodiment of her lived experience, a testament to the resilience, systems and support she wishes she had during her own caregiving journey.

As a coach and author, Andrea is determined to empower caregivers, helping them find clarity, balance and strength, proving that <u>they don't have to walk this path alone</u>.

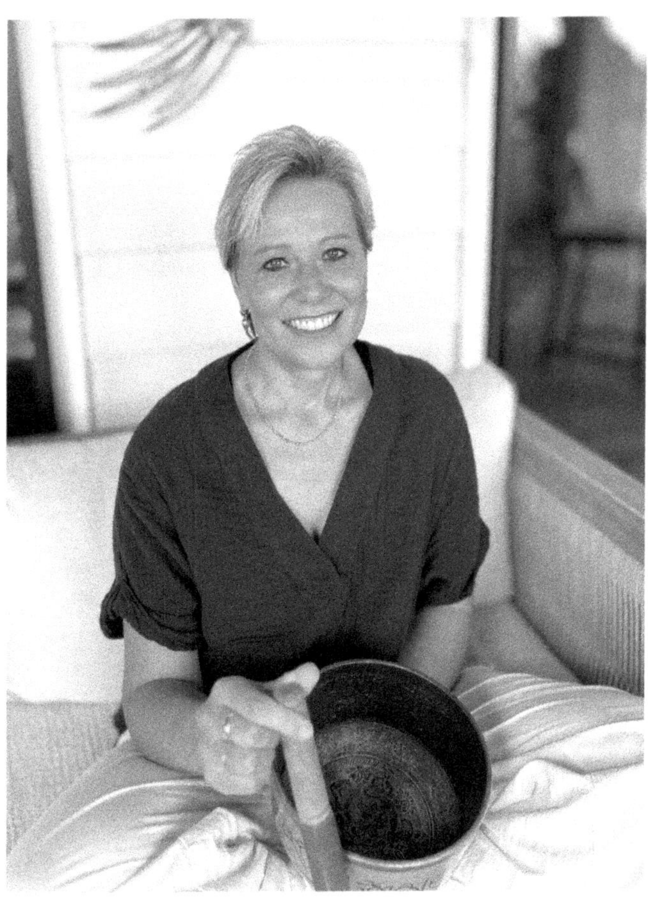

Acknowledgements

This book would not have been possible without the love, patience and support of my family.

To my husband, Colin, my rock and my greatest supporter – thank you for holding everything together while I was deep in the writing process. Your unwavering support, from taking care of the household to giving me space to create, has meant everything to me. Having you by my side to bounce ideas off, to keep me grounded and to lift me up when I needed it most has been invaluable. I am deeply grateful for the balance we share, harmonising our masculine and feminine energies as we navigate life's challenges together.

To my daughter, Jess and her fiancé, Jake and my twin boys, Kaden and Will, your encouragement kept me going when writer's block hit or when I doubted whether I would ever finish this book. Your belief in me, your constant nudges to keep pushing forward and your ability to remind me why I started this journey in the first place have meant the world.

To my dad and my sister, you were both part of the ripple effect that shaped my caregiving journey. Standing side by side as we cared for Mum, we shared moments of love, strength and unwavering dedication.

The bond we had, love and the resilience she inspired in all of us, became a profound part of my life. She was the glue that held us all together and when she passed, it was heartbreaking. Yet, through that loss, I found the courage and determination to build *A1 Quality Care*, with your constant support and belief in me, turning my personal experience into a mission to support others walking the caregiving path.

From the depths of my heart, thank you all! I love you!

This book is not just mine – it belongs to everyone who has been part of my journey.

References

American Psychological Association (2023). Retrieved from https://www.apa.org/ – *Understanding the benefits of social sharing in mental health recovery.*

Australian Bureau of Statistics (2022). *Survey of Disability, Ageing and Carers: Summary of Findings.* Retrieved from https://www.abs.gov.au/statistics/health/disability/disability-ageing-and-carers-australia-summary-findings/2022

Australian Government – Home Care Packages Program. *Guide to Aged Care Services and Support.* Retrieved from https://www.myagedcare.gov.au/home-care-packages

Cancer Council Australia. *Practical Support and Resources for Families Affected by Cancer.* Retrieved from https://www.cancer.org.au

Carers Australia. *Respite Care, Advocacy, and Caregiver Support Services.* Retrieved from https://www.carersaustralia.com.au

Carers Australia (2020). *Caring in Australia: A National Survey of Caregivers.* Retrieved from https://www.carersaustralia.com.au/wp-content/uploads/2020/10/Caring-in-Australia-Survey-2020.pdf

Deloitte Access Economics. *The Economic Value of Informal Care in Australia*. Retrieved from https://www2.deloitte.com/au/en/pages/economics/articles/economic-value-informal-care-Australia-2020.html

Dementia Australia. *Support, Helplines, and Resources for Dementia Caregivers*. Retrieved from https://www.dementia.org.au

Department of Health and Aged Care (Australia). *Aged Care Programs and Respite Services for Older Australians*. Retrieved from https://www.health.gov.au

Journal of Behavioural Medicine (2022). *Impact of Long-Term Caregiving on Mental Resilience*. Retrieved from https://link.springer.com/article/10.1007/s10865-022-00234-5

National Disability Insurance Agency (NDIA). *Managing the NDIS and Providing Support for People with Disabilities*. Retrieved from https://www.ndis.gov.au

National Disability Insurance Agency (NDIA), Local Area Coordinators (LACs), and My Aged Care (MAC). *Government-Funded Caregiving Programs and Support Services*. Retrieved from https://www.ndis.gov.au/understanding/what-ndis and https://www.myagedcare.gov.au

National Disability Insurance Scheme (NDIS). *Participant Guidelines and Funding Support*. Retrieved from https://www.ndis.gov.au/participants

National Institute for Health Research (2022). *Caregiver Burnout and Mental Health Study*. Retrieved from https://www.nihr.ac.uk/documents/caregiver-burnout-and-mental-health-study-2022/

Occupational Health and Safety (OH&S) Regulations. *Guidelines for Workplace and In-Home Safety.* Retrieved from https://www.safeworkaustralia.gov.au/

Speech Pathology Australia. *Best Practices in Communication for Caregivers.* Retrieved from https://www.speechpathologyaustralia.org.au/SPAweb/Resources_for_the_Public/Carers_and_Family_Members/

3 Offers With Calls to Action

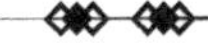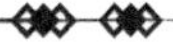

1. Build Your Own Caregiving Systems

If this book opened your eyes, this program will change your life. You've seen how structure can transform caregiving – but knowing it and doing it are two different things. That's where the *Build Your Own Caregiving System* program comes in.

This self-paced, online mastermind guides you step by step to build a system that suits *you*, your loved one and your lifestyle. With done-for-you templates, practical checklists, and expert insights, you'll stop firefighting and start feeling in control.

Guided videos walk you through each step, and fortnightly check-ins with Andrea ensure you're supported with expert advice and real-world perspective.

No more guesswork. No more overwhelm. Just a clear path forward – on your terms, with help when you need it most.

Explore the program today at www.a1-quality-care.com

2. One-on-One Coaching – Reclaim Your Life, While Still Caregiving

You're more than a caregiver – you're a whole person with dreams, goals, and a life that matters, too. Whether you're feeling burnt out, stuck in survival mode, or simply wondering *what's next*, my oneon-one coaching gives you the space to breathe, reflect and rebuild.

Together, we'll refine your caregiving journey and create personalised strategies that bring more balance to your day-to-day. You'll learn how to care with intention *while carving out time for your own needs, goals and growth*. Because being there for someone else shouldn't mean losing yourself.

Book a free strategy session today at www.a1-quality-care.com

3. A Transformational Experience – Reset and Reconnect at a Caregivers Retreat

Sometimes the most powerful way to care for others is to pause and care for yourself. *The Caring Heart Retreats* in Australia and Bali aren't just a getaway – they're a soul-deep reset. Designed exclusively for caregivers, these immersive retreats offer you space to breathe, reflect, and *transform*.

Surrounded by calm, beauty, and a like-minded community, you'll be guided through restorative workshops, pampering sessions, mindfulness practices, and practical strategies to simplify your caregiving journey.

Return home recharged, rebalanced and ready to face your role with renewed clarity, strength and heart.

Learn more about upcoming retreats at www.a1-quality-care.com

Speaker Bio

Andrea Entwistle is a caregiving coach, author and speaker with over 20 years of experience in the disability industry. Dedicated to helping caregivers find balance, resilience and support in their roles Andrea combines her personal caregiving journey with professional expertise to empower others.

As the founder of *A1 Quality Care*, she provides structured support, practical resources and coaching for caregivers who want to thrive – not just survive.

Through her workshops, retreats and online programs, Andrea has guided countless caregivers toward creating sustainable systems that reduce stress and prioritise self-care.

She believes that caregiving should not mean losing yourself in the process and she passionately teaches practical strategies to help caregivers build systems, establish boundaries and reclaim their own well-being.

Andrea is available for keynote speaking, workshops and caregiver training to help organisations, communities and individuals reshape the way caregiving is approached.

For speaking inquiries or to learn more, visit *www.a1-quality-care. com* or email Andrea at *admin@a1-quality-care.com*

Notes